Theory in a
Nutshell

Theory in a
Nutshell

SECOND EDITION

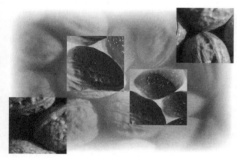

A practical
guide to
health
promotion
theories

Don Nutbeam
Elizabeth Harris

The **McGraw·Hill** Companies

Sydney New York San Francisco Auckland
Bangkok Bogotá Caracas Hong Kong
Kuala Lumpur Lisbon London Madrid
Mexico City Milan New Delhi San Juan
Seoul Singapore Taipei Toronto

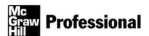

Reprinted 2004, 2005, 2007, 2008, 2009

First published 1999
Text © 2004 Don Nutbeam and Elizabeth Harris
Illustrations and design © 2004 McGraw-Hill Australia Pty Ltd
Additional owners of copyright are acknowledged on the Acknowledgments page.

National Library of Australia Cataloguing-in-Publication data:

Nutbeam, Don.
Theory in a nutshell: a guide to health promotion theory.

2nd ed.
Includes index.
ISBN 978 0 074 71332 7

1. Health promotion. 2. Health planning. I. Harris, Elizabeth. II. Title.

613

Published in Australia by
McGraw-Hill Australia Pty Ltd
Level 2, 82 Waterloo Road, North Ryde NSW 2113
Acquisitions Editor: Meiling Voon
Production Editor: Rosemary McDonald
Editor: Rosemary McDonald
Associate Editor: Thu Nguyen
Proofreader: Tim Learner
Indexer: Diane Harriman
Designer (cover and interior): Jan Schmoeger/Designpoint
Illustrator: Alan Laver, Shelly Communications
Typeset in 10/12 pt ITC Giovanni Book by Jan Schmoeger/Designpoint
Printed on 80 gsm woodfree by RR Donnelley, China.

The *McGraw-Hill* Companies

Contents

Preface   vii
Acknowledgments   ix
Introduction   xi

Chapter 1: Theory   1

What is a theory?   1
The use of theory   2
Single theory or multiple theories?   6
Further reading   9

**Chapter 2: Theories on health behaviour and health
behaviour change: individual characteristics**   10

The health belief model   10
The theories of reasoned action and planned behaviour   14
The transtheoretical (stages of change) model   16
Social cognitive theory   19
Summary   22
Further reading   23

**Chapter 3: Theories on change in communities and
communal action for health**   25

Diffusion of innovation theory   26
Community organisation and community building   30
Summary   36
Further reading   37

Chapter 4: Models for communication to bring about behaviour change 39

Communication–behaviour change model 39
Social marketing 42
Summary 47
Further reading 47

Chapter 5: Models for change in organisations and for the creation of health-supportive organisational practice 49

Theories of organisational change 50
Models of intersectoral action 53
Summary 58
Further reading 59

Chapter 6: Models for the development of healthy public policy 61

A framework for making healthy public policy 61
Evidence-based policy making to promote health 64
Impact assessment and health impact assessment 69
Summary 73
Further reading 73

Conclusion: Theory in practice 75

Index 77

Preface

Not all health promotion programs are equally successful in achieving their aims and objectives. Experience tells us that programs are most likely to be successful when the determinants of a health problem or issue are well understood, where the needs and motivations of the target population are addressed, and the context in which the program is being implemented has been taken into account. The use of theory can help achieve a better fit between problem and program.

Although many health promotion projects and programs are developed and implemented without overt reference to theory, there is substantial evidence from the literature on health promotion to suggest that the use of theory will significantly improve the chances of success in achieving predetermined program objectives. The use of theory can help in the planning and delivery of programs in several ways. Theory can:

- help us understand better the nature of the problem being addressed;
- describe and explain the needs and motivations of the target population;
- explain or make propositions concerning how to change health status, health-related behaviours and their determinants; and
- inform the methods and measures used to monitor the problem and the program.

Theory helps to achieve a better fit between problem and program.

This book is intended to provide practitioners and students of health promotion with an overview of several of the most influential theories and models which have guided health promotion practice in the recent past, and remain influential in the present.

In each case, an explanation of the main elements of the theory is provided, followed by a commentary on its relative strengths and weaknesses, and some idea on how it can be related to the real world.

Through this book we hope to demonstrate that, when used prudently, theories can greatly enhance the effectiveness and sustainability of health promotion programs.

> The use of theory can help achieve a better fit between problem and program.

Acknowledgments

Several people have contributed to the development of the second edition of this book. We would particularly like to acknowledge the contribution of the work of Karen Glanz. Her textbook on theory, research and practice is a major resource for students and is referred to regularly in this book. Her publication, *Theory at a Glance,* was a model for this book and the inspiration for the title.

In the preparation of this revised edition we would like to acknowledge the contribution of James Morrison who assisted with the review of recent literature, Clive Blair-Stevens for his contribution to the section on health impact assessment, and Mark Harris and Peter Sainsbury for their useful reviews of this revised edition.

Introduction

This book reflects the range of activities that are currently being undertaken by health promotion practitioners. It starts with an examination of theories that explain health behaviour and health behaviour change by focusing on individual characteristics. Four theories that have been influential on health promotion practice are discussed, namely the health belief model, the theory of reasoned action, the transtheoretical (stages of change) model, and social cognitive theory.

What emerges from these overviews is that while these theories contribute substantially to our understanding of individual behaviour, unless behavioural theories are put into the broader context in which the individual is living, many factors that influence health will remain unexplained.

It is now well recognised that the capacity and opportunities for individuals to bring about change to their health can be significantly affected by the competence of the community in which they live to address issues beyond the control of any one individual. This means that we need to understand theories that help explain how the capacity of communities can be strengthened and how new ideas can best be introduced into communities. Correspondingly, theories of community organisation and community building are discussed as well as the diffusion of innovation theory.

In order to raise awareness and engage individuals, groups and communities in taking action to promote health, a number of theories and models have been developed to guide ways in which health messages can be most effectively communicated and acted upon. The two most influential—communication–behaviour change theory and social marketing—are discussed. Both have provided very practical and effective guidance to those developing mass communication strategies. However, their impact is often limited if relevant organisational structures do not support or facilitate the changes they seek to bring about.

Many organisational structures (sometimes referred to as settings) can have both direct and indirect impacts on people's health. These settings, such as schools, worksites and recreational venues, are places where people spend a great deal of time. Such settings directly influence health through the services and programs that they provide to individuals and communities, and through the opportunities and constraints they place on individuals and health-related behaviour (e.g. facilities for physical activity, restrictions on smoking). Less directly, such settings influence health by providing access to social support, or, more negatively, as a source of stress and conflict. They can also have indirect impacts through, for example, planning regulations by councils, and income support policies of the government. In this context this book looks at two models that help practitioners to understand how to influence change within organisations and enable them to work effectively together. These are discussed as theories of organisational change and a model for understanding intersectoral action.

Finally, this book looks at the emerging field of healthy public policy and models that are being developed to understand how policy can be influenced and changed to promote health. These include a framework for making healthy public policy, evidence-based policy making to promote health and health impact assessment.

This second edition includes revisions and updates to all sections, as well as new sections on community organisation and community building, evidence-based policy making to promote health, and health impact assessment.

> Unless behavioural theories are put into the broader context in which the individual is living, many factors that influence health will remain unexplained.

Table I.1 Summary of models presented in this book

Area of change	Theories or models
Theories that explain health behaviour and health behaviour change by focusing on the individual	Health belief model Theory of reasoned action Transtheoretical (stages of change) model Social cognitive theory
Theories that explain change in communities and communal action for health	Diffusion of innovation Community organisation and community building
Theories that guide the use of communication strategies for change to promote health	Communication–behaviour change model Social marketing
Models that explain changes in organisations and the creation of health-supportive organisational practices	Theories of organisational change Models of intersectoral action
Models that explain the development and implementation of healthy public policy	A framework for making healthy public policy Evidence-based policy making to promote health Impact assessment and health impact assessment

Chapter 1
Theory

What is a theory?

A fully developed theory would explain:

- **the major factors that influence the phenomenon of interest**, for example, those factors which explain why some people are regularly active and others are not;
- **the relationship between these factors**, for example, the relationship between knowledge, beliefs, social norms and behaviours such as physical activity; and
- **the conditions under which these relationships do or do not occur**: the *how, when* and *why* of hypothesised relationships, for example, the time, place and circumstances which, predictably, lead to a person being active or inactive.

A commonly used definition of a theory is:

Systematically organised knowledge applicable in a relatively wide variety of circumstances devised to analyse, predict, or otherwise explain the nature or behaviour of a specified set of phenomena that could be used as the basis for action.[1]

Most health promotion theories come from the behavioural and social sciences. They borrow from various disciplines such as psychology, sociology, management, consumer behaviour and marketing. Such diversity reflects the fact that health promotion practice is not only concerned with the behaviour of individuals but also with the ways in which society is organised and the policies and organisational structures that underpin social organisation.

---

1   Van Ryn, M., Heany, C.A. (1992), 'What's the use of theory?', *Health Education Quarterly*, 19, 3, pp. 315–330.

Many of the theories commonly used in health promotion are not highly developed in the way suggested in the definition above, nor have they been rigorously tested when compared, for example, with theory in the physical sciences. For these reasons many of the 'theories' included in the book are more accurately referred to as theoretical frameworks or models.

The use of theory

The potential of theory to guide the development of health promotion interventions is substantial. There are several different planning models that are used by health promotion practitioners. Internationally, the best known of these planning models is the **precede/proceed** model developed by Green and Kreuter. Several variations of this approach have also been produced (see Further Reading at the end of this chapter for more information).

> The potential of theory to guide the development of health promotion interventions is substantial.

In each case these planning models and guidelines follow a structured sequence including planning, implementation and evaluation stages. Reference to different theories can guide and inform practitioners at each of these stages.

Figure 1.1 presents a health promotion planning and evaluation cycle, indicating the various stages in the planning, implementation and evaluation of a health promotion program.

Defining the problem

Identification of the parameters of the health problem to be addressed may involve drawing on a wide range of epidemiological and demographic information, as well as information from the behavioural and social sciences, and knowledge of community needs and priorities. Here, different theories can help us identify what should be the focus for an intervention.

Specifically, theory can inform choice of the elements we should consider as the focus for the intervention. For example, the health belief model and theory of reasoned action help identify individual characteristics, beliefs and values that are associated with different health behaviours and may be amenable to change.

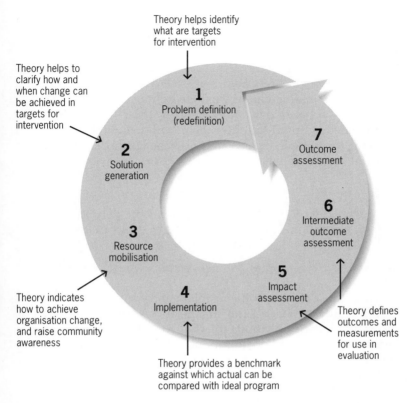

Figure 1.1 Health promotion planning and evaluation cycle

Similarly, organisational change theory helps identify key elements of organisations which may need to be changed and are amenable to change.

Planning a solution

The second stage in the cycle indicates the need for the analysis of potential solutions, leading to the development of a program plan which specifies the objectives and strategies to be employed, as well as the sequence of activity. Theory is at its most useful here in providing guidance on how and when change might be achieved in the target population, organisation or policy. It may also prompt ideas which would not have routinely occurred to us.

Different theories can help us understand the methods we could use as the focus of our interventions, specifically by improving understanding of the processes by which changes occur in the target variables (i.e. people, organisations and policies), and by clarifying the means of achieving change in these target variables. For example, social cognitive theory helps explain the relationship between personal observation and experience, social norms, and the influence of different external environments and their impact on individual behaviour. The insights to these relationships that are provided by social cognitive theory will help in the design of a program, for example, by indicating how changes to the environment or social norms can have an impact on health behaviour.

> Theories also inform decisions on the timing and sequencing of our interventions in order to achieve maximum effects.

Thus, those theories which explain and predict individual and group health behaviour and organisational practice, as well as those that identify methods for changing these determinants of health behaviour and organisational practice, are worthy of close consideration in this phase of planning.

Some theories also inform decisions on the timing and sequencing of our interventions in order to achieve maximum effects. For example, stages of change theory and diffusion of innovation theory provide guidance on the sequence and timing of activities with individuals and communities.

Mobilising resources for implementation

Once a program plan has been developed, the first phase in implementation is usually directed towards generating public and political interest in the program, mobilising resources for program implementation, and building capacity in partner organisations through which the program may operate (e.g. schools, worksites, local government). Models of intersectoral action, which help us understand how to build partnerships, and organisational change theory, which indicates how to influence organisational policy and procedures, are particularly useful here, as is communication–behaviour change theory that can guide the development of media-based, awareness-raising activities.

Implementation

The implementation of a program may involve multiple strategies such as education and advocacy. Here, the key elements of theory can provide a benchmark against which the actual selection of methods and sequencing of an intervention can be considered in relation to the theoretically ideal implementation of programs.

In this way the use of theory helps us to explain success or failure in different programs, particularly by highlighting the possible impact of differences between what was planned and what actually happened in the implementation of the program. It can also assist in identifying the key elements of a program that can form the basis for disseminating successful programs.

Evaluation

Health promotion interventions can be expected to have different levels of impact and different effects over time. Impact evaluation represents the first level of outcome evaluation of a program. The adoption of theory in the planning of programs can provide guidance on the measures that can be used to assess the success of programs. For example, where theory suggests that the target of interventions is to achieve change in knowledge and self-efficacy, or changes in social norms or organisational practices, measurement of these changes becomes the first point of evaluation. Such impact measures are often referred to as health promotion outcomes.

Intermediate outcome assessment is the next level of evaluation. Theory can also be used to predict the intermediate health outcomes that are sought from an intervention. Usually these are considered in terms of modification of individual behaviour or modifications to social, economic and environmental conditions that determine health or influence behaviour. Several theories, such as the health belief model and social cognitive theory, predict that changes to health promotion outcomes will lead to change in health behaviour.

Health outcome assessment refers to the end point outcomes of an intervention in terms of change in physical or mental health status, in quality of life, or in improved equity in health within populations. Definition of these final outcomes will be based on theoretically predicted relationships between changes.in the determinants of risk (intermediate health outcomes) and final health outcomes.

Figure 1.1 indicates that each of these evaluation stages leads back to a redefinition of priority problems and solutions, hence the concept of a cycle of planning and evaluation.

Table 1.1 summarises the tasks and potential of theory to support the planning, execution and evaluation of health promotion programs.

Table 1.1 The use of theory in program planning and evaluation

Planning phase	Task	Possible use of theory
Problem identification and prioritisation	Clarify major health issues for a defined population, and prioritise in terms of the potential for effective intervention	Clarify what should be the target elements of an intervention, such as individual beliefs, social norms or organisational practices
Planning a solution	Develop a program plan which specifies program objectives, strategies and the sequence of activity	Guidance on how, when and where change can be achieved in the target elements of a program
Mobilising resources for implementation	Generate public and political support, build the capacity of partner organisations and secure resources	Guidance on how to build partnerships, raise public awareness and foster organisational development
Implementation	Execute the program as planned, utilising multiple strategies (as appropriate to the program objectives)	Provide a benchmark against which the actual implementation can be compared with the theoretically ideal
Evaluation	Assess the impact and outcome of the program according to predefined program objectives	Define outcomes and measurements which could be used at each level of evaluation

Single theory or multiple theories?

Theories are not a series of static pronouncements that can be applied to all issues in all circumstances. In health promotion some of the theories that have been used have been extensively refined and developed in the light of experience. The range and focus of theories has also expanded over the past two decades from a focus on the modification of individual behaviour, to recognition of the need to influence and change a broad range of social, economic and environmental factors that influence health alongside individual behavioural choices.

Thus, contemporary health promotion operates at several different levels:

- individual
- community
- organisational settings
- public policy and practice

Choosing the right approach is moderated by the nature of the problem, its determinants and the opportunities for action.

Programs which operate at multiple levels, such as those that draw upon combinations of the strategies described in the Ottawa Charter for Health Promotion, are most likely to address the range of determinants of health problems in populations, and thereby have the greatest effect.

For example, a program to improve uptake of immunisation will generally be more effective when based on a combination of interventions. These might include:

- education to inform and motivate individual parents to immunise their children;
- facilitation of community debate to change perceptions concerning the safety and convenience of immunisation;
- changes to organisational practice to improve notification systems;
- provision of more conveniently located clinics; and
- financial incentives for parents and doctors.

It follows that no single theory dominates health promotion practice, and nor could it, given the range of health problems and their determinants, the diversity of populations and settings, and differences in available resources, skills and opportunity for action among practitioners.

Depending on the level of intervention (individual, group, or organisation), the type of change (simple, one-off behaviour, complex behaviour, organisational or policy change), different theories will have greater relevance, and provide a better 'fit' with the problem. In many cases it will be possible and appropriate to combine different models and theories to achieve goals across the spectrum of health promotion actions.

None of the theories or models presented in this book can simply be adopted as the answer to all problems. Most often, we benefit by drawing upon more than one of the theories presented here to match the multiple levels of the program response being contemplated.

> In many cases it will be possible and appropriate to combine different models and theories to achieve goals across the spectrum of health promotion actions.

To be useful and relevant, the different models and theories have to be readily understood, and genuinely capable of application to a wide variety of real-life conditions of practice.

Although we are constantly reminded that 'there is nothing so practical as a good theory',[2] many of us remain somewhat suspicious of the capacity of intervention theories to provide the guidance necessary to develop an effective intervention in a complex environment.

Karen Glanz offers a commonsense summary of how to judge a good fit between a theory or combinations of theories and the problem you are trying to address. It is:

- logical;
- consistent with everyday observations;
- similar to those used in previous successful program examples you have read or heard about; and
- supported by past research in the area or related areas.

Ultimately, theories and models are simplified representations of reality—they can never include or explain all of the complexities of individual, social or organisational behaviours. However, while the use of theory alone does not guarantee effective programs, the use of theory in the planning, execution and evaluation of programs will enhance the chances of success. One of the greatest challenges for practitioners is to identify how best to achieve a fit between the issues of interest and established theories or models which could improve the effectiveness of a program or intervention. This book is intended to assist you in meeting this challenge.

---

2   ibid.

Further reading

Glanz, K., Lewis, F.M., Rimer, B.K. (2002), *Health Behavior and Health Education: Theory, Research and Practice*, 3rd edition, Jossey-Bass, San Francisco, California.

Green, L.W., Kreuter, M.W. (1999), *Health Promotion Planning: An Educational and Environmental Approach*, Mayfield, Mountain View, California.

Nutbeam, D. (2001) 'Effective Health Promotion Programmes', in Pencheon, D., Guest, C., Meltzer, D., Muir Gray, J.A. *Oxford Handbook of Public Health Practice*, Oxford University Press, Oxford.

Chapter 2
Theories on health behaviour and health behaviour change: individual characteristics

One of the major roots of contemporary health promotion can be found in the application of health psychology to health behaviour change. Evidence for this can be seen in the phenomenal growth in the discipline of health psychology and the evolution of the concept of behavioural medicine. This discipline has been a significant influence in the USA, where for several decades researchers have sought to explain, predict and change health behaviour by the development and application of theories and models evolving from the disciplines of psychology and the hybrid social psychology. Four of the most influential are described below.

The health belief model

The health belief model is one of the longest established theoretical models designed to explain health behaviour by better understanding beliefs about health. It was originally articulated to explain why individuals participate in public health screening and immunisation programs and has been developed for application to other types of health behaviour.

At its core, the model suggests that the likelihood of an individual taking action related to a given health problem is based on the interaction between four different types of belief. Figure 2.1 summarises the different elements of the model. The model predicts that individuals will take action to protect or promote health if:

- they perceive themselves to be susceptible to a condition or problem;
- they believe it will have potentially serious consequences;
- they believe a course of action is available that will reduce their susceptibility, or minimise the consequences; and

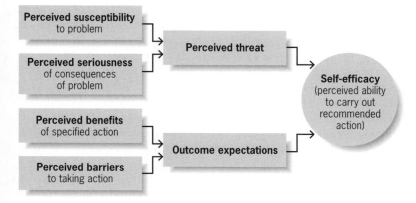

Figure 2.1 Health belief model: major components and linkages

- they believe that the benefits of taking action will outweigh the costs or barriers.

Later refinements have acknowledged the important modifying factors, particularly those associated with personal characteristics and social circumstances as well as the impact of more immediate cues for action, such as media publicity or personal experience. Added to this analysis is the concept of self-efficacy—that is, the belief in one's competency to take appropriate action—as a further factor influencing the strength of the model in predicting behaviour change.

For example, if we consider the application of this model to the prevention of Human Immunodeficiency Virus (HIV) infection, in order to adopt behaviours that minimise risk of infection, individuals need to:

- believe that they are at risk of HIV infection;
- believe that the consequences of infection are serious;
- receive supportive cues for action which may trigger a response (such as targeted media publicity);
- believe that risk minimisation practices (such as safe sex or abstinence) will greatly reduce the risk of infection;
- believe that the benefits of action to reduce risk will outweigh potential costs and barriers, such as reduced enjoyment, and negative reactions of partner and/or community; and
- believe in their ability to take effective action, such as following and maintaining safe-sex practice.

Although it was not always consciously done, many of the early public education campaigns concerning HIV/AIDS prevention took this approach. Initially this was done by seeking to persuade people that they were at risk and by emphasising the deadly nature of Acquired Immune Deficiency Syndrome (AIDS). Later, as the epidemic developed, public education campaigns focused more on the efficacy of safe sex (particularly the use of condoms) in minimising the risk of infection and on improving people's confidence to use condoms. The use of theory can be very useful in thinking about what information you may need to collect from a target group before a program is developed.

An early review of findings[1] from interventions using the health belief model provided persuasive evidence to support the usefulness of the model in predicting why individuals adopted (or failed to adopt) different health behaviours. In the thirty years following this publication the model has been widely adopted as a planning tool for health education programs intended to promote greater compliance with preventive health behaviours and health care recommendations.

> The use of theory can be very useful in thinking about what information you may need to collect from a target group before a program is developed.

Subsequent reviews have provided mixed evidence of success, but have helped to refine our understanding of the best application of the model. Overcoming perceived barriers to successful action was identified as the most important element of the model. Perceived susceptibility and perceived benefits were also recognised as important.

In a review of the model in 1984[2] the authors point to the limitations of the health belief model in predicting and explaining health behaviour:

> The health belief model is a psychosocial model; as such it is limited to accounting for as much of the variance in an individual's health

---

1 Becker, M.H. (ed.) 'The Health Belief Model and Personal Health Behavior', *Health Education Monography,* 2, pp. 324–473.

2 Janz, N.K., Becker, M.H. (1984), 'The Health Belief Model: A Decade Later', *Health Education Quarterly,* 11, pp. 1–47.

behaviour as can be explained by their attitudes and beliefs. It is clear that other forces influence health actions as well.

These 'other forces' include social, economic and environmental conditions, which significantly shape the barriers to action that are fundamental to the model. For example, limited access to health care services and/or resources can, of course, greatly impede effective health actions, and will in turn influence the individual's perceptions of barriers and benefits, which are integral to the model.

If we go back to the example of the HIV/AIDS public education campaigns, some of the limitations of the health belief model become apparent. The lack of accessible sexually transmissible diseases services, the cost or availability of condoms, pressures on some groups (such as commercial sex workers) to act in unsafe ways in order to keep customers, can all work against people adopting behaviours that they know will reduce their risk of infection. Individual behaviour and the beliefs that influence it need to be seen in this wider context.

> Changes in knowledge and beliefs will almost always form part of a comprehensive health promotion program and the health belief model provides an essential reference point in the development of messages.

Commentary

The health belief model has been found to be most useful when applied to behaviours for which it was originally developed, particularly traditional preventive health behaviours such as screening and immunisation. It has been less useful in guiding interventions to address more long-term, complex and socially determined behaviours such as alcohol and tobacco use.

The model's great use is in the relatively simple way in which it illustrates the importance of individual beliefs about health, and the relative costs and benefits of actions to protect or improve health. Three decades of research have indicated that promoting change in those beliefs can lead to changes in health behaviour that contribute to improved health status. Changes in knowledge and beliefs will almost always form part of a comprehensive health promotion program, and the health belief model provides an essential reference point in the development of messages to improve knowledge and change beliefs, especially messages designed for use in the media.

The theories of reasoned action and planned behaviour

The theory of reasoned action was developed by Ajzen and Fishbein to explain human behaviour that is under 'voluntary' control. A major assumption underlying the theory is that people are usually rational and will make predictable decisions in well-defined circumstances. The model is predicated on the assumption that intention to act is the most immediate determinant of behaviour, and that all other factors influencing behaviour will be mediated through behavioural intention.

The top part of Figure 2.2 shows how behavioural intentions are thought to be influenced by attitudes towards behaviours and subjective norms. Attitudes, in this case, are determined by the belief that a desired outcome will occur if a particular behaviour is followed, and that the outcome will be beneficial to health (similar to perceived benefits and barriers in the health belief model). This part of the figure summarises Ajzen and Fishbein's original theory of reasoned action.

Subjective norms, in this case, relate to a person's beliefs about what other people think they should do (normative beliefs) and by an individual's motivation to comply with those other people's wishes. These social influences vary in strength related to the degree to which the individual values social approval by a particular group.

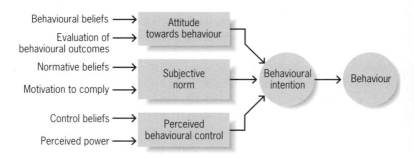

Figure 2.2 Theory of planned behaviour: major components and linkages

For example, if an individual who smokes feels that most people do not smoke and that most of their valued friends and colleagues want them to quit, then it is most likely that the person would consider that there is a norm which favours quitting smoking.

Intentions to act are thus jointly determined by attitudes and subjective norms. Put simply, the theory predicts that a person is most likely to intend to adopt, maintain or change a behaviour if they believe the behaviour will benefit their health, is socially desirable and feels social pressure to behave in that way. According to the theory, if these beliefs and social pressures are strong enough, this intention to behave will subsequently be transferred into behaviour. By influencing beliefs and exerting social pressure, behaviours can be changed or maintained.

Ajzen and Fishbein take this analysis one step further by indicating that it is the short-term consequences of behaviours that are the most powerful in predicting attitudes towards behaviour and that subjective norms are most affected by significant others. These significant others might include, for example, a person's valued peers, and media celebrities and sports stars who act as role models.

Ajzen and others have developed this theory further and have added perceived behavioural control as a third influence on behavioural intentions. This recognises that a person's intentions will become significantly greater if they feel they have greater personal control over a behaviour—a concept closely allied to self-efficacy—and that this is also mediated by their perceived power in relation to a given situation. In making this adjustment Ajzen recognised that there are many factors beyond the immediate control of individuals that will shape their ability to behave in a desired way. As a consequence, Ajzen proposed changing the name of the theory to theory of planned behaviour.

The theory can be very useful in identifying what information you may need to collect from a target group before a program is developed. It highlights the need to understand the beliefs of the group about the issue, who they see as affecting these beliefs and their behaviour, and what they perceive as the barriers to taking actions that might promote their health.

For example, in developing a heart health education program in a minority ethnic community it will be important to understand what they believe are the causes of heart disease and the actions that they feel they can confidently take to reduce their risk. It will also be important to identify who are the significant others that shape decisions that could reduce the risk of heart disease. If the program was trying to change eating patterns it may be the oldest woman in the household or the eldest son who has the most influence over the family's diet.

Ajzen and Fishbein's original model was widely applied to the development of programs to reduce uptake of smoking among youth during the 1980s. These programs recognised that information on the consequences of smoking should emphasise the short-term negative consequences, such as the affect on appearance and the financial cost, as opposed to long-term negative consequences such as lung cancer and heart disease. Such programs also recognised the role of significant others in shaping decisions to smoke, by utilising peer leaders in smoking education programs and by recruiting acknowledged role models for young people. More recently the theory has been applied to the development of programs to reduce risks of transmission of HIV and other sexually transmitted diseases.

Commentary

The results of the smoking education programs referred to above were weaker than expected, resulting in the modifications to the theory described above. Subsequent applications of the model have demonstrated its usefulness in identifying factors that influence health behaviour that may become targets for intervention. Past failures of programs based on the theory of reasoned action have highlighted not only the difficulty of translating models that predict behaviour change into successful health promotion interventions, but also the dangers of choosing to focus on just a few elements in a complex model. The model is most successfully applied when all elements are considered in an intervention. Its proponents stress the importance of conducting in-depth interviews to identify the most important beliefs that are relevant to the behaviour concerned. As with the health belief model, the theory of reasoned action provides valuable insight into key factors that influence behaviour, and provides a strong indication of the importance of perceived social norms and understanding of short-term consequences in shaping health behaviour.

The transtheoretical (stages of change) model

This model was developed by Prochaska and DiClimente to describe and explain different stages of change which appear to be common to most behaviour change processes. The model has two basic dimensions which describe both the different stages of change, and processes of change relevant to the different stages. The model is based on the premise that <u>behaviour change is a process, not an event,</u> and that individuals have varying levels of motivation or readiness to change.

Five basic stages of change have been identified:

1. **precontemplation**: this describes individuals who are not even considering changing behaviour, or are consciously intending not to change;
2. **contemplation**: the stage at which a person considers making a change to a specific behaviour;
3. **determination, or preparation**: the stage at which a person makes a serious commitment to change;
4. **action**: the stage at which behaviour change is initiated; and
5. **maintenance**: sustaining the change and achievement of predictable health gains. **Relapse** may also be the fifth stage.

A sixth stage of **termination** has also been identified as appropriate to some behaviours, especially addictive behaviours. This represents a stage where individuals have no temptation and high self-efficacy in relation to the changed behaviour, as though they had never acquired the habit (such as smoking) in the first place.

People appear to move in a predictable way through these stages, although some move more quickly than others, and some get 'stuck' at a particular stage. A person's confidence in their ability to change and overcome perceived barriers, and 'decisional balance' (a person's relative weighting of the pros and cons of making change) are among the factors identified as influencing progression between stages.

The model is circular rather than linear, as people can enter or exit at any point, and it applies equally to people who self-initiate change and those who are responding to external stimuli such as advice from health professionals or health campaigns.

This model has applications at both the individual and the broader program level. For example, for health practitioners, such as general practitioners, this model provides a useful way of thinking about the advice that they are trying to give patients and may help to reduce the frustration they feel when their advice is not taken. The model provides a way of establishing if their patient wants to change, assists in identifying barriers to making change, and recognises that relapsing is a common problem in any change process (see Table 2.1).

Table 2.1 Use of the transtheoretical model by general practitioners to promote weight control among patients

Stages of change	Process of change	GP action
Precontemplation	Consciousness-raising	Discusses with the patient the health problems associated with being overweight and the feasibility of weight loss
Contemplation	Recognition of the benefits of change	Discusses with the patient the potential benefits to them of proposed change—illustrates success
Determination or preparation	Identification of barriers	Assists patient in identifying potential barriers they may face and how these can be addressed—emphasises the relative benefits
Action	Program of change	Works out a plan for weight loss and exercise with the patient and monitors closely
Maintenance	Follow-up and continuing support	Organises routine follow-up and discusses with patient the likelihood of relapse

From a program planning perspective, the model is particularly useful in indicating how different processes of change can influence how programs or activities are staged. Prochaska and colleagues have identified several processes of change that have been most consistently useful in supporting movement between stages. These different processes are more or less applicable at different stages of change. For example, consciousness-raising may be most useful among precontemplators who may not be aware of the threat to their health that their behaviour poses, whereas communication of the benefits of change and illustration of the success of others in changing health behaviour may be most important for those contemplating change. Once the change process has been initiated at the action stage, social support and stimulus control (for example, by avoiding certain situations, or having environmental supports in place) are more important.

By matching stages of behavioural change with specific processes the model specifies how interventions could be organised for different populations with different needs and in different circumstances. The stages of change model provides important advice on the need to research the characteristics of the target population and the need not to assume that all people are at the same stage and the need to organise interventions sequentially to address the different stages that will be encountered.

Commentary

The stages of change model has quickly become an important reference point in health interventions on a range of issues including smoking cessation, physical activity, weight control and use of mammography services. Apart from the obvious advantage in health promotion of focusing on the change process, the model is important in emphasising the range of needs for intervention in any given population, the changing needs of different populations and the need for sequencing of interventions to match different stages of change. It illustrates the importance of tailoring programs to the real needs and circumstances of individuals rather than assuming an intervention will be equally applicable to all.

Although the transtheoretical model has been proposed as a model which serves as an umbrella for other theories that guide health promotion practice, its strong roots in behavioural psychology and primary application in clinical settings with individuals makes this assessment somewhat optimistic. It may be best considered as an approach to defining needs and intervening to improve the health of individuals or groups.

Social cognitive theory

Social cognitive theory has evolved from social learning theory and is one of the most widely applied theories in health promotion because it addresses both the underlying determinants of health behaviour and methods of promoting change. Social cognitive theory has evolved with input from several researchers over the past fifty years but, in terms of its application to health promotion, the most influential writer has been Albert Bandura.

Social learning theory was built on an understanding of the interaction that occurs between an individual and their environment. Early psychosocial research tended to focus on the way in which an environment shapes behaviour, by making it more or less rewarding to behave in particular ways. For example, if at work there is no regulation on where people are able to smoke cigarettes, it is easy to be a smoker. If regulations are in place it is more difficult, and as a consequence most smokers smoke less and find such an environment more supportive for quitting.

Social cognitive theory indicates that the relationship between people and their environment is more subtle and complex. For example, in circumstances where a significant number of people are non-smokers and are assertive about their desire to restrict smoking in a given environment, even without formal regulation, it becomes far less rewarding for the individual who smokes. They are then likely to modify their behaviour. In this case the non-smokers have influenced the smoker's perception of the environment (referred to as situation in the theory) through social influence.

Bandura refers to this principle as reciprocal determinism. It describes the way in which an individual, their environment and behaviour continuously interact and influence each other. Understanding of this interaction and the way in which (in the example) modification of social norms can impact on behaviour offers an important insight into how behaviour can be modified through health promotion interventions. For example, seeking to modify social norms regarding smoking is considered to be one of the most powerful ways of promoting cessation among adults.

Added to this basic understanding of the relationship between behaviour and the environment, Bandura has also determined that a range of personal cognitive factors form a third part to this relationship, affecting and being affected by specific behaviours and environments. Of these cognitions, three are particularly important. First is the capacity to learn by observing both the behaviour of others and the rewards received for different patterns of behaviours (observational learning). For example, some young women may observe behaviours, such as smoking, by people who they regard as sophisticated and attractive, i.e. role models. If they observe and value the rewards that they associate with smoking, such as sexual attractiveness or a desirable self-image, then they are more likely to smoke themselves—their expectancies in relation to smoking are positive. Such an understanding further reinforces the importance of taking account of peer influences and social norms on health behaviour, and of the potential use of role models in influencing social norms.

Second is the capacity to anticipate and place value on the outcome of different behaviour patterns (referred to as expectations). For example, if you believe that smoking will help you lose weight, and place great value on losing weight, then you are more likely to take up or to continue smoking. This understanding emphasises the importance of understanding personal beliefs and motivations underlying different behaviours, and the need to emphasise short-term and tangible benefits or negative effects of behaviours. For example, young people have been shown to respond far more negatively to the short-term effects of smoking (bad breath, smelly clothes) than to any long-term threat posed to health by lung cancer or heart disease.

Third, Bandura's work emphasises the importance of belief in your own ability to successfully perform a behaviour (referred to as self-efficacy). Self-efficacy is proposed as the most important prerequisite for behaviour change and will affect how much effort is put into a task and the outcome of that task. The promotion of self-efficacy is thus an important task in the achievement of behaviour change. Bandura has proposed that both observational learning and participatory learning (e.g. by supervised practice and repetition) will lead to the development of the knowledge and skills necessary for behaviour change (behavioural capability) and are powerful tools in building self-confidence and self-efficacy.

As is the case in the interaction between behaviour and the environment, the relationship between these personal characteristics, behaviour and the environment is reciprocal and dynamic. For example, a young woman who is quitting smoking may be very confident (high self-efficacy) in her ability to abstain at work where smoking is banned and none of her workmates smoke, but she may be less confident when she goes out with her friends who are heavy smokers. Thus self-efficacy is both behaviour-specific and situation (environment) specific.

This explicit acknowledgment of the dynamic and reciprocal relationship between an individual, their behaviour and the environment avoids overly simple solutions to health problems that focus on behaviour in isolation from the social environment. An understanding of the characteristics of the person assists in the creation of educational interventions to alter the knowledge, understanding, beliefs and skills which affect observational learning, outcome expectations and self-efficacy. Such interventions are intended to improve the capacity of an individual to behave in a desired way. Understanding the way in which the physical and social environments act to provide incentives or disincentives for different behaviours points to ways of constructing interventions to modify the environment to further support healthy behaviours and provides opportunities to change. Recognition that the importance of factors relating to the person and the environment will vary with different behaviours adds a further depth to the development of an intervention.

Commentary

Taken as a whole, social cognitive theory provides a comprehensive theoretical basis for health promotion programs. It recognises the fundamental importance of individual beliefs, values and self confidence in determining health behaviour. It also explicitly identifies the importance of social norms and cues, and environmental influences on health behaviour, and the continuous interaction between these variables. Social cognitive theory provides practical direction on how to modify these influences. In this sense it provides an important bridge between this section of the book and the sections which follow on community mobilisation, organisational change and public policy development.

The model also suggests a role for the health practitioner which may be less overtly interventionist than the ways implied by the models described earlier. The health worker becomes a 'change agent', facilitating change through modification of the social environment and the development of personal competencies that enable individuals to act to improve their health.

It also assists in understanding the levels or layers at which a health promotion program may need to work. For example, in trying to reduce the number of young women who take up smoking it may be as important to address the issue of body image as to provide information on the short- and long-term consequences of smoking.

Not surprisingly, a review of health promotion literature in the past decade reveals a large number of health promotion interventions that combine educational programs with modification of the social and physical environments based on social cognitive theory. This continuous 'field testing' adds further confidence to the usefulness of this theory to guide practice.

Summary

This overview of theories that explain health behaviour and health behaviour change by focusing on the individual provides important guidance on major elements of health promotion programs. Taken together the theories and models described above emphasise:

- the importance of knowledge and beliefs about health. All of the theories and models presented in this chapter imply a central role for health education and refer to individual knowledge about health. They emphasise the importance of personalising health information, such that it is more immediately relevant to an individual, and the short-term consequences of behaviours.
- the importance of self-efficacy: the belief in one's competency to take action. The development of personal skills and self-confidence that create self-efficacy, through personal observation, supervised practice and repetition, is central to success in each of the models presented.
- the importance of perceived social norms and social influences related to the value an individual places on social approval or acceptance by different social groups. The influence of social role models, family and peer groups is emphasised here.
- the importance of recognising that individuals in a population may be at different stages of change at any one time.
- limitations to psychosocial theories that do not adequately take account of socioeconomic and environmental conditions that significantly shape access to services and resources.
- the importance of shaping or changing the environment or people's perception of the environment as an important element of programs.

Further reading

The health belief model

Harrison, J.A. et al. (1992), 'A Meta-analysis of Studies of the Health Belief Model', *Health Education Research*, 7, 1, pp. 107–116.

Janz, N.K., Becker, M.H. (1984), 'The Health Belief Model: A Decade Later', *Health Education Quarterly*, 11, pp. 1–47.

Janz, N.K., Champion, V.L., Strecher, V.J. (2002), 'The Health Belief Model', in Glanz, K. et al. *Health Behavior and Health Education: Theory, Research and Practice*, 3rd edition, Jossey-Bass, San Francisco, California.

The theories of reasoned action and planned behaviour

Ajzen, I., Fishbein, M. (1980), *Understanding Attitudes and Predicting Social Behavior*, Prentice-Hall, Englewood Cliffs, New Jersey.

Ajzen, I. (1991), 'The Theory of Planned Behavior', *Organizational Behavior and Human Decision Processes*, 50, pp. 179–211.

Montano, D.E., Kasprzyk, D. (2002), 'The Theory of Reasoned Action and Theory of Planned Behavior', in Glanz, K. et al. *Health Behavior and Health Education: Theory, Research and Practice*, 3rd edition, Jossey-Bass, San Francisco, California.

The transtheoretical (stages of change) model

Prochaska, J.O., DiClimente, C.C. (1984), *The Transtheoretical Approach: Crossing Traditional Boundaries of Therapy*, Dow Jones Irwin, Homewood, Illinois.

Prochaska, J.O. et al. (1994), 'Stages of Change and Decisional Balance for Twelve Problem Behaviors', *Health Psychology*, 13, pp. 39–51.

Prochaska, J.O., Redding, C.A., Evers, K.E. (2002), 'The Transtheoretical Model and Stages of Change', in Glanz, K. et al. *Health Behavior and Health Education: Theory, Research and Practice*, 3rd edition, Jossey-Bass, San Francisco, California.

Social cognitive theory

Bandura, A. (1986), *Social Foundations of Thought and Action: A Social Cognitive Theory*, Prentice Hall, Englewood Cliffs, New Jersey.

Bandura, A. (1995), *Self-efficacy in Changing Societies*, Cambridge University Press, New York.

Baranowski, T., Perry, C.L., Parcel, G.S. (2002), 'How Individuals, Environments and Health Behaviour Interact', in Glanz, K. et al. *Health Behavior and Health Education: Theory, Research and Practice*, 3rd edition, Jossey-Bass, San Francisco, California.

Chapter 3
Theories on change in communities and communal action for health

Many of the factors that influence health and health-related behaviour can be traced to the social structures and the wider social environment. Many of these influences are most obvious when working in, and with, the community. People feel connected to their community and it is often possible to take action to improve health by working in community settings. For this reason, understanding the ways in which social structures impact on health and developing skills in working with communities is important in contemporary health promotion practice.

In the past, the 'community' has been seen simply as a collection of individuals or a venue through which it is possible to reach large numbers of people to bring about larger scale health behaviour changes than might be typical through more individual forms of intervention. Many early 'community-based' programs such as the Stanford Heart Programs in the 1970s could be characterised this way. However, in contemporary health promotion practice, communities are viewed as dynamic systems with inherent strengths and capabilities that can be influenced and supported in ways that will improve health.

This section considers three theories or models for working with communities:

1. introducing new ideas into communities (diffusion of innovation);
2. identifying key approaches by organisations and workers to bring about change in local communities (community organisation); and
3. making communities more central in decisions about their futures (community building).

> Understanding the ways in which social structures impact on health and developing skills in working with communities is important in contemporary health promotion practice.

Diffusion of innovation theory

The systematic study of the ways in which new ideas are adopted by communities has its roots in the examination of the ways in which new agricultural technologies were introduced into both developed and developing countries. Over time these studies have been expanded to the introduction of new ideas, practices and technologies in other disciplines, including health. The most widely acknowledged researcher of the diffusion process in relation to health innovation is Everett Rogers who has synthesised experience from hundreds of case studies to develop the theory of innovation diffusion and applied it in a wide variety of settings.

Diffusion is defined as:

the process by which an innovation is communicated through certain channels over time among members of a social system.

An innovation is defined as:

an idea, practice or object perceived as new by an individual.[1]

In this case, it is important to emphasise the perceived newness of an idea, regardless of its first use or discovery. If an idea is new to an individual, then it is an innovation.

Diffusion of innovation theory has evolved through examination of the processes by which innovations are communicated and adopted (or not). The work of Rogers and colleagues has identified five general factors that influence the success and speed with which new ideas are adopted in communities. Understanding of these factors is central to the application of diffusion theory to health promotion innovations. The factors are:

1. the characteristics of the potential adopters;
2. the rate of adoption;

---

1   Rogers, E.M. (1983), *Diffusion of Innovations*, 3rd edition, Free Press, New York.

3. the nature of the social system;
4. the characteristics of the innovation; and
5. the characteristics of change agents.

Some individuals and groups in society tend to be quicker to pick up new ideas than others. Others in the community tend to be more suspicious of change and slow to respond to 'new-fangled' ideas. Stereotypically, farmers are cautious in their response to innovation.

Rogers uses a system of classifying different adopters into categories according to the time it takes for adoption to occur. Innovators are those two to three per cent of the population who are quickest to adopt new ideas. However, they may be regarded as fickle, and are less likely to be trusted by the majority in the community. Early adopters are those ten to fifteen per cent of the population who may be more mainstream within the community, but are the most amenable to change, and have some of the personal, social or financial resources to adopt the innovation. The early majority are those thirty to thirty-five per cent of the population who are amenable to change and have become persuaded of the benefits of adopting the innovation. The late majority are those thirty to thirty-five per cent of the population who are sceptics and are reluctant to adopt new ideas until such time as the benefits have been clearly established. The laggards are the final ten to twenty per cent of the population who are seen to be the most conservative and in many cases actively resistant to the introduction of new ideas. As indicated by the different percentages for each group, Rogers suggests that their distribution in a population matches the 'normal' probability distribution curve.

> It is essential to know the community with whom you are working and what is likely to influence their response to new ideas.

From this simple classification it is possible to see how age, disposable income and exposure to the media are, for example, all important variables which will define the different types of 'adopter' and influence the speed of uptake of innovations. As ever, it is essential to know the community with whom you are working and what is likely to influence their response to new ideas.

Rogers has also shown that the cumulative number of adopters can be plotted against time to produce the S-shaped curve shown in Figure 3.1. Rogers emphasises that different innovations take vastly different time periods to introduce to the majority of the target population, and, in some cases, will never reach the entire population. The increasing difficulty of influencing late adopters and the residual group of laggards translates into diminishing returns on effort in health programs and needs to be recognised in the planning and evaluation of programs.

What becomes obvious from an examination of this model is the importance of identifying ways of speeding up the adoption process. Factors in different social systems greatly influence the rate of adoption of new ideas. For example, 'traditional' communities, such as rural communities, where a population is more homogenous and inward looking, will generally take longer to adopt any innovation, partly because their exposure to innovations is less common and partly because their cultures may have evolved in such a way as to be more suspicious of change.

In other social groups, change and innovation are much more common, particularly in societies with well-developed communication systems. As a consequence these populations are more experienced in dealing with innovation and better equipped to support the process of diffusion.

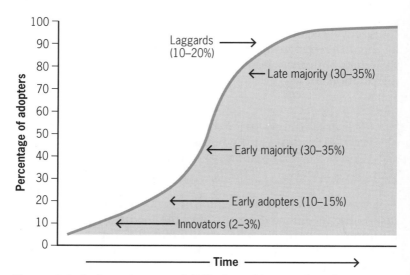

Figure 3.1 S-shaped curve of diffusion of innovations in communities

Analysis of programs has led to identification of characteristics of innovations that have been consistently associated with successful adoption. These include:

- compatibility with prevailing socioeconomic and cultural values of the adopter. For example, if a change in diet is being advocated in a particular community, it is more likely to be adopted if the food is based on traditional food sources.
- clarity of the relative advantage of the innovation compared with current practices including perceived cost effectiveness, as well as usefulness, convenience and prestige—is the food (such as fresh fruit and vegetables) conveniently available at a price that people can afford?
- the simplicity and flexibility of the innovation. Those that require simple actions and that can be adapted to different circumstances are more likely to be successful—is the food simple to prepare and consume, and no new cooking methods are required?
- the reversibility and perceived risk of adoption. Innovations perceived as high risk or involving an irreversible change in practice are less likely to be adopted—no new cooking utensils need to be bought.
- observability of the results of adopting an innovation to others who may be contemplating change. For example, there are stories in local news sources showing the impact of a changed diet on a person's life.

Although it is rare for any innovation to meet all of these criteria, an understanding of these characteristics can help in the development of programs as well as in the identification of implementation problems. For example, in trying to influence the diet of Aboriginal communities in remote parts of Australia it is important to recognise that more fresh food in the diet: assumes that there are ways of buying, storing and cooking fresh foods; may involve more preparation time than older methods; and may require significant changes in existing food consumption patterns.

Finally, Rogers identifies the importance of the change agent who facilitates the adoption of change in a population. This may be an independent person working with a community to introduce an innovation, or may be a person from the community who is operating to facilitate change. Allied to this, community members can act as role models for other adopters. Selection of appropriate role models, particularly from among community leaders, can help accelerate the rate of adoption in a community.

There is a clear coincidence of ideas between Rogers' studies of the diffusion process and Bandura's social change theory. The latter emphasises the central role of social modelling in learning about innovation and in providing motivation for its adoption.

Diffusion theory is not only applicable to the introduction of new ideas into communities, but can also be considered in relation to organisations. This is of great importance in the context of health promotion, both in terms of creating supportive environments for health, and in the long-term maintenance of programs. The same type of analysis as that described above can be applied to organisations. Various studies have examined, for example, the introduction of innovations to schools and health-care settings.

Commentary

Diffusion of innovation theory has been developed and tested in a wide variety of settings and for many different purposes. It provides an excellent diagnostic tool for analysing how and why populations respond to the introduction of new ideas, emphasising the importance of systematic research and planning to maximise the chances of success. The coincidence of themes with social cognitive theory further emphasises the importance of role modelling and social reinforcement of change.

Diffusion theory is of particular importance in guiding programs that are devoted to maximising the adoption of projects which have previously been shown to be effective, and is a critical tool in the transfer of evidence-based practice.

However, there are limitations to the theory especially in relation to the concept of laggards. It may not only be conservative attitudes and resistance to change that prevent them from adopting new behaviours, but also a lack of resources or other structural barriers. An uncritical adoption of the notion of limited returns in trying to change the remaining twenty per cent of a population may reinforce inequalities that are not necessarily due to individual choice.

Community organisation and community building

Working with local communities or communities of interest (such as gay groups, indigenous and ethnic minority groups, or groups representing people with a disability) has been a central strategy for health promotion workers to improve health or address specific problems. Community organisation has been defined as the process by which community groups are helped to identify common problems or goals, mobilise resources, and in other ways develop and implement strategies for reaching the goals they have collectively set.

At the community level, several strategies for community organisation have evolved over many years. The most widely recognised typology to describe these approaches was developed by Rothman who identified three models of practice: locality development, social planning and social action.

Locality development emphasises community participation and methods that promote ownership of issues. This approach to community mobilisation is strongly process-oriented, focusing on consensus, cooperation and building community capacity to define and solve community problems. In this model the role of a professional practitioner is as a catalyst and facilitator rather than a leader.

By contrast, social planning is more task-oriented and expert-driven. It is based on a rational–empirical approach to problem definition and involves professional 'planners' in the development of solutions. The role of the practitioner in this model is one of 'fact gatherer and analyst' and program implementer. This model reflects epidemiological analysis of health problems, and a tightly organised, professionally determined and planned programmatic response.

The third model, social action, is characterised by both a concern for processes which build community capacity and with the achievement of tangible change in a community in favour of the most disadvantaged. Achieving such change inevitably involves shifts in power relationships and resources. The practitioner role in such a model is one of advocate and mediator on behalf of disadvantaged groups.

> Social action is characterised by both a concern for processes which build community capacity and with the achievement of tangible change in a community in favour of the most disadvantaged.

In proposing these models, Rothman made it clear that none of the models is mutually exclusive, but rather that efforts at community mobilisation will tend towards one or another of the three categorisations. The use of the term 'locality development' has been criticised because it implies that this model of community organisation is applicable only to geographically defined communities. The alternative and the more commonly used term is community development.

Community organisation conceived of in these ways is a useful way of linking individuals, community groups, workers and leaders in a community. It provides a framework within which interventions can be planned and implemented at several levels. For example, developing a program to reduce childhood injury in a community may involve a mix of locality development (working with local community groups to share ideas on the nature of the problem and discussion of possible solutions), social planning (introduction of traffic calming devices into the local environment), and social action (local advocacy for safe pedestrian crossings).

Theories and models of community development continue to evolve, in part in reaction to the perceived limitations of Rothman's typology. Key criticisms concern the extent to which these early models of community organisation were too problem-based (seeking solutions to predefined problems), and had their roots in approaches to development that were significantly dependent upon outside technical expertise and professional support. These approaches fail to capture the importance of building capacity within communities and, related to this, to foster community empowerment.

At the heart of the distinction between Rothman's construct of community organisation and what Minkler refers to as community building are concepts of empowerment and capacity building. Empowerment is defined by Minkler as a social action process in which individuals, communities and organisations gain mastery over their lives in the context of changing their social and political environment to improve equity and quality of life. Minkler and others argue that empowerment becomes a fundamental resource that can be used in a variety of situations to improve opportunities for health.

Rissel has proposed an empowerment 'continuum' that helps to differentiate between stages in the development of empowerment. In this model the stages can apply equally to individuals and communities:

- Health professionals can work with people in ways that increase an individual's confidence that they have the capacity to act in ways that will bring about change.
- Involvement in mutual support groups, self-help or action groups builds and expands social networks and provides

opportunities for further personal development. During this process an individual may become critically aware of the wider social forces that are acting on them and their community. Participation in and the influence of community groups is important in both psychological and community empowerment. It is often how people learn new skills that they may be able to use in other situations and also builds the capacity of communities to solve problems.

- As the community becomes more empowered it will work on specific issues, link with other groups to take wider action and ultimately may engage in collective political or social action.

Goodman and colleagues define community capacity as the characteristics of communities that affect their ability to identify, mobilise and address social and public health problems. They help to develop our understanding of the multiple dimensions of community capacity. For example, they see community capacity reflected in the number and skills of local leaders to take up issues, the levels of trust and willingness to work together within communities and the ability of local communities to freely share information and to solve problems in innovative and effective ways. They also point out that the capacity of communities is built up over time and so it is important to understand the history of the community and how this has shaped its current circumstances.

Bush, Dower and Mutch have further developed the dimensions of community capacity and developed a way of identifying and monitoring community capacity. This can assist health promotion practitioners working with local communities to identify current levels of capacity and to identify ways in which community capacity can be further developed. They stress the importance of build capacity to address particular issues or needs—it is something that needs to be developed by 'doing'.

They have identified four broad domains of community capacity:

1. **Network Partnerships** are the relationships between groups and organisations within a community or network. This includes both the comprehensiveness and the quality of the relationships, that is, are all of the significant groups and organisations involved and what is the nature of their involvement.
2. **Knowledge transfer** is the development, exchange and use of information within and between the groups and organisations within a network or community.

3. **Problem solving** is the ability of the groups and organisations within the network or community and of the network or community itself to use well-recognised methods to identify and solve problems that arise in the development and implementation of an activity or program.
4. **Infrastructure** refers to the level of investment in a network by the groups and organisations making up the network. This includes both tangible and non-tangible investments, such as investment in policy and protocol development, social capital, human capital and financial capital.

Bush and his colleagues developed their framework based on an extensive review of the literature and case studies. They believe that a key component of building capacity is also building sustainability. Increases in community capacity that are also accompanied by increases in infrastructure are seen as being most sustainable.

When thinking about working in and with communities it is important that practitioners reflect on the extent to which their work is focused on problems that have been identified by the community or by people or services outside the community. For example, service providers may decide that the biggest issue in a community is coronary heart disease while the community itself may be more concerned with the high levels of crime in the area. Negotiating these different perspectives will be important in planning effective action.

Figure 3.2 shows how health promotion practitioners can have an important role in each of these types of activity. In general, the approaches that are based on an assessment of community needs, engage and empower communities, and contribute to increased community capacity are most likely to achieve sustainable, long-term outcomes.

Commentary

Unlike the theories and models of health behaviour change at the individual level, community organisation does not lend itself so comfortably to highly structured study and to comprehensive theory development. It is not easy to plan or control. However, community organisation approaches as described by Rothman and others provide a practical framework through which health promotion workers can think about ways in which they may work most effectively with geographically defined communities or with communities of interest. There is a growing body of literature that reports on the

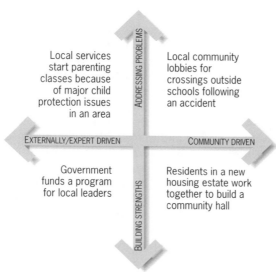

Figure 3.2 Dimensions of community organisation and capacity building

evaluation of complex, community based interventions. Over time, this will improve our ability to account for the high variation in context (time, place, issue, person) that influences the course and effectiveness of community interventions.

Community organisation approaches enable health promotion workers to address the underlying social determinants of health. Such methods encourage the involvement of communities in defining the problems that they face and in taking action to address them and enhances the likelihood that changes brought about within communities can be sustained.

Although empowerment of individuals, groups and communities is implied in community organisation approaches it is not necessary for local people to define the problem to be addressed or to take major responsibility for action. Several critics feel that community organisation models often take a 'deficit' approach to thinking about communities—focusing only on problems rather than community strengths. As a consequence, such approaches may fail to recognise and build on the existing strengths in communities.

Despite these perceived limitations there are many examples of situations when the use of the community organisation framework will provide practical guidance on how health promotion workers can work with local communities and service providers to tackle significant health problems.

Community building based on empowerment is conceptually attractive, but difficult to deliver in practice. Empowerment of individuals and communities is a time intensive process, one that requires a high level of trust and commitment between those involved and a willingness by the health promotion worker to relinquish power. This is especially challenging when working with the most disenfranchised and marginalised groups in society.

Despite a high level of interest in concepts of community building, community capacity, and the related concept of social capital, these approaches have limitations. For example, there is a risk that focusing on the need to build community capacity may indirectly pass responsibility to communities to solve their own problems, regardless of the root causes. There is an underlying assumption that the most important social forces impacting on people can all be changed at a local level, however, this will not always be the case. In addition, by working with the most visible leaders in local communities, health promotion workers can further empower the empowered and continue to marginalise those who are disenfranchised.

Summary

This overview of approaches to working in and with communities to improve health demonstrates the breadth of action that is characteristic of current health promotion thinking. This ranges from approaches that are strongly based on building community competency and control as an integral element to achieving improvements in health, through to those that are overtly health-goal directed and that draw on a sophisticated understanding of how to speed the diffusion of predesignated ideas in communities.

The diffusion of innovation theory provides guidance on how to introduce new health practices or services into a community. The framework of community organisation described by Rothman provides a sound foundation for working with local communities. Both help health promotion workers to define what it is they are intending to achieve and provides practical guidance on how this can be done. They help us to think about why, how and in what way local communities may be involved in health promotion programs.

The (re)emergence of empowerment and capacity building as drivers in community development reminds us of the importance of seeing communities and their individual members as having strengths and capacities that need to be recognised and developed. Each of these approaches has to be considered on its merits and placed in the context (people, place and time) in which a program is being developed.

Several themes can be drawn from this overview:

- The diffusion of new ideas and practices through communities does not occur by chance, and can be significantly influenced by effective change agents in communities. The importance of effective mass communication and role modelling is emphasised in this process.
- A focus on working at the community level has the advantage of dealing more overtly with the social, economic and environmental determinants of health that have their origins in local conditions.
- It provides opportunities for empowering individuals and communities to take action that will improve their health.
- Skills for health include not only those required to take personal actions that will protect and support health but also the ability and capacity to act collectively.
- Reducing inequalities in health may involve investing additional resources in building the capacity of those communities that are most disadvantaged to actively participate in and guide programs to improve their health.

Further reading

Diffusion of innovation theory

Oldenberg, B. & Parcel, G.S. (2002), 'Diffusion of Innovations', in Glanz, K. et al. *Health Behavior and Health Education: Theory, Research and Practice*, 3rd edition, Jossey-Bass, San Francisco, California.

Parcel, G.S., Perry, C.L., Taylor, W.C. (1990), 'Beyond Demonstration: Diffusion of Health Promotion Innovations', in Bracht, N. (ed.) *Health Promotion at the Community Level*, Sage, Newbury Park, California.

Rogers, E.M. (1983), *Diffusion of Innovations*, 3rd edition, Free Press, New York.

Rogers, E.M. (2002), 'Diffusion of Preventive Interventions', *Addictive Behaviors*, 27, pp. 989–993.

Community organisation and community building

Bush, R., Dower, J., Mutch, A. (2002), *Community Capacity Index*, Centre for Primary Health Care, University of Queensland, Brisbane.

Minkler, M. (ed.) (1999), *Community Organizing and Community Building for Health*, Rutgers University Press, New Jersey.

Minkler, M. & Wallerstein, N.B. (2002), 'Improving Health through Community Organization and Community Building', in Glanz, K. et al. *Health Behavior and Health Education: Theory, Research and Practice*, 3rd edition, Jossey-Bass, San Francisco, California.

Rissell, C. (1994), 'Empowerment: The Holy Grail of Health Promotion', *Health Promotion International*, 9, 1, pp. 39–47.

Rothman, J. (2001), 'Approaches to Community Interventions', in Rothman, J., Erlich, J.L., Tropman, J.E. (eds) *Strategies of Community Interventions*, Peacock Publishers, Itascam, Illinois.

Chapter 4
Models for communication to bring about behaviour change

As has been outlined in the previous chapters, effective health promotion strategies are best developed by engaging individuals and communities in the issues to be addressed. This involves understanding the beliefs and knowledge that people have about a problem and their skills in addressing it, as well as broader community understanding of why the issue is important and how it can most effectively be tackled.

Clear communication between health promotion practitioners and those who they are trying to influence is essential. Several models of how this can best be done have emerged, and two of these are outlined below. They are the communication–behaviour change model and the social marketing model.

Communication–behaviour change model

The communication–behaviour change model was developed by McGuire to design and guide public education campaigns. It is included here because the model is based on communication inputs and outputs which are designed to influence attitudes and behaviour in similar ways to the theories and models described in earlier chapters.

> The content and form of a message can influence audience response.

The five communication inputs described by McGuire are:

1. **Source:** the person, group or organisation from whom a message is perceived to have come. The source can influence

the credibility, clarity and relevance of a message. For example, the same message delivered from a government source, by a celebrity, or from a non-government organisation will have different credibility and relevance to different target audiences.

2. **Message:** what is said and how it is said. The content and form of a message can influence audience response. For example, the use of fear or humour to communicate the same message may provoke different responses from different target audiences. Practical considerations such as length of message, form of language and tone of voice also need to be considered.

3. **Channel:** the medium through which a message is delivered. Traditionally the media include television, radio, print media (e.g. newspapers, pamphlets, posters), as well as techniques such as direct mail. More recently information technology has opened up a range of new media for use in communicating health messages, including the Internet and mobile phone text messages. Issues to be considered in selecting a channel for communication include the potential reach of different media, the cost of use and differences in the complexity of message that can be communicated through different media.

4. **Receiver:** the intended target audience. Recognising differences in audience segments and their media preferences are important in matching the right message to the right channel from the right source. Social and demographic variables, such as gender, age, ethnic background, income and location, as well as current attitudes, behaviours and media use, can all be considered as a part of this element.

5. **Destination:** the desired outcome to the communication. This may include change in attitudes or beliefs, or, more likely, changes in behaviour.

This model can be very useful in conceptualising and designing mass communication strategies. For example, in trying to highlight a men's health issue such as the risk of prostate cancer, it will be important for the source of the message to be someone respected by the men most at risk and with whom they can identify. The message will need to be portrayed in an acceptable way, for example, by using humour to portray situations men face. It will need to be communicated through media used by these men, with decisions made on which messages can best be communicated by TV, which by printed material, and which through advertisements. There will need to be some decision on who is the target group. Is it all men? What are the subgroups? How influential are 'significant others', such as partners and parents, in bringing about change? And finally what is it that the communication strategy is hoping to achieve—awareness raising or some more specific action?

The communication–behaviour change model also provides a twelve-step sequence of events, representing outputs from a communication, which link initial exposure to a communication to long-term change in behaviour. These are:

- exposure
- attention
- interest
- understanding
- skill acquisition
- attitude change
- memorisation
- recall
- decision-making
- behaviour change
- reinforcement
- maintenance.

These steps illustrate that for a communication strategy to be effective the message has to be carefully designed and delivered through an appropriate channel to reach the target audience. The population has to be exposed to the message (no mean feat in itself!), pay attention to it and understand it. Even if a message has achieved this, there are still eight more steps to the achievement of sustainable health behaviour change.

Once understood by an individual, the message must create an inclination to change, reflected in attitude change that is stored and maintained until such time as the receiver is in a position to act on that attitude change. Once the decision to change a behaviour has been made and acted on, this new behaviour needs reinforcement to be maintained.

These inputs and outputs can be put together as a matrix to illustrate the need to change the input mix depending on the targeted output. Different sources, messages and channels will be required to reach different receivers and achieve different outcomes.

Commentary

Even though this model is not based on substantial empirical testing in the same way as the health belief model and theory of reasoned action, it is based on the same general links between beliefs and perceptions, attitudes and behaviour that are illustrated by these other models.

The communication–behaviour change model shows just how difficult it can be to develop a public communication campaign, which by itself leads to sustainable behaviour change. This model provides an excellent overview of the range of issues which needs to be considered in the development of a public education campaign. Although several major public intervention programs (such as the first Stanford three-cities program in the US, which was intended to reduce the risks for heart disease in the community) have been based on this model, progressive experience in using the mass media for public communication has led to a better understanding of the advantages and limitations of media campaigns in terms of cost, reach and effect. Media campaigns are now more commonly used to influence public knowledge, attitudes and opinions as part of a more comprehensive strategy that places mass communication within a wider repertoire of interventions.

Social marketing

Social marketing evolved as a technique to influence social norms and health behaviours in the 1970s. These early approaches were based on the simple adaptation of established commercial marketing techniques for the achievement of social change. Maibach and colleagues have more recently defined social marketing as:

> A process that attempts to create voluntary exchange between a marketing organisation and members of a target market based on mutual fulfilment of self-interest.[1]

The authors go on to state that the marketing organisation uses its resources to:

- understand the perceived interests of target market members;

---

1 Miabach, E.W., Rothschild, M.L., Novelli, W.D. (2002), 'Social Marketing', in Glanz, K. et al. *Health Behavior and Health Education: Theory, Research and Practice*, 3rd edition, Jossey-Bass, San Francisco, California.

- enhance and deliver the package of benefits associated with a product, service or idea; and
- reduce barriers that interfere with the adoption or maintenance of that product, service or idea.

Target market members, in turn, expend their resources (such as money, time or effort) in exchange for the offer when it provides clear advantages over alternative behaviors. Success of the social marketing program is defined primarily in terms of its contribution to the wellbeing of target market members or to society as a whole.

This definition emphasises the importance of benefit to individuals and society. It is these benefits and the nature of the relationship between the 'buyer' (target market) and 'seller' (health organisation or practitioner) that helps to distinguish social marketing for health promotion and disease prevention from commercial marketing. Social marketing differs from commercial marketing in its intent to benefit the target population and/or society in general, rather than to benefit the marketer.

> Social marketing differs from commercial marketing in its intent to benefit the target population and/or society in general, rather than to benefit the marketer.

In commerce, marketing is designed to influence consumer choice. The marketplace exchange is the commodity or service sold and money collected. Success can be measured in the volume of these exchanges. Although improving knowledge of a product or changing attitudes and values towards the product may be a means to influence purchasing behaviour, these are not in themselves the objective of marketing.

Social marketing is also intended to influence how people think and, ultimately, how they behave. Similarly it is based on a change in behaviour with costs and benefits to the individuals concerned. Immunisation offers protection against measles; a parent considers the costs and benefits of this 'product' and decides whether or not to engage in this behaviour—whether to 'buy' immunisation. Success can be measured in the number of people who are immunised.

Although the costs may not be financial and the benefit not material, the same objective of achieving a change in behaviour is at the heart of the social marketing process. However, social marketing does differ from commercial marketing in its intent to benefit the target population and/or society in general, rather than only to benefit the marketer. Thus the relationship between the 'seller' and 'buyer' will in many cases be very different from that in commercial marketing. The definition above emphasises that this is a voluntary exchange, based on mutual fulfilment of self-interest—both parties are clearly seen to benefit, rather than one exploiting the other.

The social marketing cycle

The social marketing cycle was developed by Novelli and proposes six sequential stages to a social marketing strategy. These account for the needs of the target audience, the development and implementation of a marketing strategy to reflect those needs and tracking of audience response to the strategy.

Marketing analysis

Social marketing has a strong 'consumer' orientation, rather than a focus on selling a product or service through persuasive communication. This requires a good understanding of the priority population through market research into underlying knowledge and attitudes to the issue or service, and potential channels for communication (e.g. literacy, media use). Such market research is intended to lead to clearly defined marketing objectives and strategies for achieving them, and to allow for segmentation of different priority populations with different needs and interests. This is followed by development and testing of the marketing plan elements and subsequent implementation. For example, finding out the groups of people in which immunisation rates are lowest and exploring the reasons why some children have not been immunised.

Selecting channels and materials: the marketing mix

Marketing strategies are multifactorial and generally based on achieving a balanced mix of four major inputs, commonly referred to as the four Ps of product, price, promotion and placement.

The product is often difficult to define in a health promotion program; we are not often selling tangible goods or services, or immediate rewards for expenditure. Identifying what is 'on offer' and presenting an appropriate image for the priority population is essential. For example, in the case of immunising children it is important to distinguish between the procedure (the injection), the service offered (the visit to GP or nurse), and the health status achieved (protection against future disease) as each may have different meaning and relevance to different target populations.

The price signifies the relationship between the costs and benefits of the 'product'. The costs may be real or perceived, and may include financial (e.g. the cost of visiting the GP), social (e.g. social pressure from family to have the child immunised), or opportunity costs (e.g. taking time off work to attend a local clinic). Equally, the benefits may be real or perceived. The costs and benefits of advocated actions need to be carefully considered in relation to different population subgroups. In the case of immunisation, many parents may never have seen a child with a vaccine-preventable disease and have no real conception of what it is they are trying to prevent. Strategies to effectively communicate benefits and to reduce costs (real and perceived) have to be developed. Such an analysis is similar to the analysis of benefits and barriers described in the health belief model.

Wide ranges of techniques for promotion are used in social marketing. These include the purchased media (e.g. advertising, leaflets), non-purchased media (e.g. news coverage), sponsorship, participation events, direct selling, competitions etc. Selecting the most appropriate channel, message delivery and source for the priority population are essential for success. Such an analysis could be based on the development of inputs described by McGuire in his communication–behaviour change model.

In all forms of marketing the final step to success is in finding high access points for a defined priority population: the right placement. This critical aspect of 'access' has often been neglected in the development of health programs. For example, the use of health screening services is determined in part by the convenience of access, and the sensitivity of service providers to language barriers and different cultural and religious norms.

Achieving the right marketing mix is at the heart of the social marketing process. Failure to address any one of the four elements will reduce the chances of success, as will over-concentration on one element alone. There can be nothing more frustrating than, for example, mounting a successful campaign to promote uptake of immunisation, only to find that service providers are unable to cope with increased demands for services and stocks of vaccine are running low.

Implementation, assessment and feedback

These stages represent the management of a social marketing program and are not unique to social marketing in that sense. Monitoring the implementation of a program according to a planned schedule and monitoring its impact and effects according to predetermined objectives are a routine element to all health promotion programs. Social marketing is an iterative process, and the model is intended to account for changes in audience responses and changes in the external environment which governs the implementation process (e.g. funding and organisational structures). In this final stage, any changes to the environment are considered alongside information from the evaluation to guide the evolution of the next cycle.

Commentary

Social marketing offers a sophisticated model for achieving defined behavioural objectives in identified priority populations. It is less a theory in the formal sense defined earlier than a planning model for health promotion. The social marketing wheel illustrates the cyclical nature of the marketing process, offering a systematic, research-based process for problem solving which includes the planning, implementation and feedback loops that are common to such models. It offers an opportunity to integrate elements of different theories (such as the health belief model and the communication–behaviour change model), using each to advantage in a complete program model.

It is particularly useful because it encourages creative approaches to the analysis of issues and to the development of programs, especially in relation to the development of channels for communication and messages. For example, social marketing has encouraged us to look outside typical analyses of populations (e.g. age, sex, social class) in order to define consumer groups based on their media consumption or family structure. Social marketing has supported experimentation with the use of a wide repertoire of different intervention methods including mass communication, sponsorship of events and competitions, all of which have been effectively used for health promotion. Social marketing also supports a strong consumer focus in the development and delivery of programs.

However, it would be a mistake to imagine that social marketing simply involves taking marketing strategies from the commercial sector and applying them to achieve health goals. The 'product' in terms of improved health or protection against disease is often intangible, the 'price' usually not financial. Health promotion programs also operate from a different philosophical and moral base from many traditional marketing campaigns that are driven by financial gain. In such circumstances the marketing techniques to achieve sustained mass behaviour change are a great deal more complex than promoting a tangible product based on financial exchange in the commercial marketplace.

Summary

Both of the models presented in this section provide insight and guidance on the strengths and weaknesses of mass communication for health promotion. The social marketing theory provides a substantial model for planning and executing an integrated mass communication campaign.

Both models illustrate the limits of different forms of mass communication in producing substantial mass behaviour change, but also illustrate the important role of mass communication in raising awareness of health issues and in securing public and political support for different forms of health promotion intervention. Both models indicate the complexity of mass communication and illustrate:

- the importance of adequate market research to define issues, segment target populations and to test communication ideas;
- the need to match the source, message, medium and receiver in developing mass communication campaigns;
- the need to consider a wide range of different methods of communication, and different venues and settings (promotion and placement) in the development of mass communication campaigns; and
- the importance of basing the evaluation of mass communication campaigns on realistically defined outcomes.

Further reading

Communication–behaviour change model

Atkin, C., Wallack, L. (1990), *Mass Communication and Public Health*, Sage, Newbury Park, California.

Egger, G., Donovan, R., Spark, R. (1993), *Health and the Media: Principles and Practices for Health Promotion*, McGraw-Hill, Sydney.

McGuire, W.J. (1989), 'Theoretical Foundations of Campaigns', in Rice, R.E., Atkin, C. (eds) *Public Communication Campaigns*, Sage, Newbury Park, California.

Social marketing

Andreasen, A.R. (1995), *Marketing Social Change: Changing Behavior to Promote Health, Social Development and the Environment*, Jossey-Bass, San Francisco, California.

Kotler, P., Roberto, E.L. (1989), *Social Marketing: Strategies for Changing Public Behaviour*, Free Press, New York.

Ling, J.C., Franklin, B.A., Lingstead, J.F., Gearon, A.N. (1992), 'Social Marketing: Its Place in Public Health', *Annual Review of Public Health*, 13, pp. 341–362.

Miabach, E.W., Rothschild, M.L., Novelli, W.D. (2002), 'Social Marketing', in Glanz, K. et al. *Health Behavior and Health Education: Theory, Research and Practice*, 3rd edition, Jossey-Bass, San Francisco, California.

Chapter 5
Models for change in organisations and for the creation of health-supportive organisational practice

Health promotion practitioners are interested in influencing organisations for a number of reasons:

- we are usually employed by organisations and have an interest in ensuring that our own organisation is able to support the work that we are doing;
- we are interested in influencing the activities or policies of other organisations who have an influence on the health of the population; and
- we have to find ways to enable organisations to work together to promote the health of the population.

Goodman and colleagues have succinctly described the problems and potential rewards of facilitating change in organisations:

> Organisations are layered. Their strata range from the surrounding environment at the broadest level, to the overall organisational structure, to the management within, to work groups, to each individual member. Change may be influenced at each of these strata, and health promotion strategies that are directed at several layers simultaneously may be most durable in producing the desired results. The health professional who understands the ecology of organisations and who can apply appropriate strategies has a powerful tool for change.[1]

---

1 Goodman, R.M., Steckler, A., Kegler, M.C. (2002), 'Mobilising Organizations for Health Enhancement: Theories of Organizational Change', in Glanz, K. et al. *Health Behavior and Health Education: Theory, Research and Practice*, 2nd edition, Jossey-Bass, San Francisco, California.

Unlike many of the theories and models described above, the application to health problems of existing theories concerning organisational change is far less developed and analysed, or systematically tested. In this chapter we look at models of how organisational change can be applied to organisations, and models that describe and explain how organisations can work together—often referred to as intersectoral action.

> The health professional who understands the ecology of organisations and who can apply appropriate strategies has a powerful tool for change.

Theories of organisational change

Most of our understanding of how to produce organisational change has come from the development of management theory (and practice). This body of theory and knowledge has developed to explain organisational change for a variety of purposes, often in relation to improving organisational performance. This literature provides useful clues as to how to analyse different organisational settings and how to plan for change. Often these theories identify a number of stages or phases of change within organisations.

Goodman and colleagues propose a four-stage model for organisational change that is applicable to health promotion practice. They emphasise the importance of recognising the different stages, and of matching strategies to promote change in each of the stages, similar in structure to the stages of change theory and diffusion of innovation theory in previous chapters. The four stages are:

- Stage 1: **awareness raising**. This stage is intended to stimulate interest and support for organisational change at a senior level by clarifying health-related problems in the organisational environment and identifying potential solutions. For example, awareness raising may involve senior managers and administrators in the education system becoming concerned about tobacco control and recognising the potential role to be played by the education system. These 'senior level administrators' are likely to be the most influential in decisions to adopt new policies and programs in an organisation. If they are convinced of the importance of a problem and the need for a solution involving their organisation, then the strategy moves to the next stage.

- Stage 2: **adoption**. This stage involves planning for and adoption of a policy, program or other innovation that addresses the problem identified in Stage 1. This includes the identification of resources necessary for implementation. In larger organisations, this stage will often involve a different level in the management structure—the gatekeepers—who are more closely associated with the day-to-day running of an organisation. In the example above this could involve school principals and senior teachers responsible for school curricula and organisation. Ideally, this stage will involve negotiation and adaptation of intervention ideas in order to make them compatible with the circumstances of individual organisations. This element of adaptation is often essential to the adoption of change in organisations, but frequently missed by those attempting to disseminate new ideas through organisations.

- Stage 3: **implementation**. This stage is concerned with technical aspects of program delivery, including the provision of training and material support needed for the introduction of change. In the example above, this could involve classroom teachers, as they will be most directly responsible for the introduction of change. This phase may involve training and the provision of resource support to foster the successful introduction of a program. This capacity building is essential for the successful introduction and maintenance of change in organisations. Many policy initiatives fail at this point because too little attention is given to the detail of the implementation process, and too little support is offered to the individuals at the level at which implementation takes place in an organisation.

- Stage 4: **institutionalisation**. This stage is concerned with the long-term maintenance of an innovation once it has been successfully introduced. Senior administrators again become the leading players, by establishing systems for monitoring and quality control, including continued investment in resources and training.

In developing their ideas, Goodman and colleagues have drawn upon several established theories that describe and explain organisational change and development. These theories have evolved to include environmental influences and how the norms and values of entire organisations are transformed. The related concepts of organisational climate and culture and organisational capacity need to be recognised and understood in the execution of a staged approach to organisational change described above.

Organisational climate is often referred to as the 'personality' of organisations—meaning those characteristics that distinguish one organisation from another, that are based on the collective perceptions of those that live and work in that environment, and that influence their behaviour. For example, some schools are more or less authoritarian in their relations with students; public services are more or less customer focused; some work sites value and reward staff loyalty more than others. These characteristics are seen as dynamic, and are affected by a wide range of variables, many of which are external to the organisation. The term organisational culture is often used interchangeably with climate, but is distinguished as meaning a set of values and assumptions about an organisation that have formed over time, are more stable and are more resistant to change. Both organisational climate and culture can influence an organisation's capacity to function effectively, and in turn may determine the outcome of efforts to bring about change in organisations. Organisational capacity can also be seen in more practical terms such as having appropriately trained personnel, effective management systems and sufficient resources. Organisational climate, culture and capacity are all important variables that will influence the pace and extent of change that may be achieved through the stage process described above.

Achieving organisational change may involve interventions designed to alter the organisational climate and to build organisational capacity. This capacity building is an important element of effective health promotion practice. Hawe and colleagues have defined capacity building as:

> the development of sustainable skills, structures, resources and commitment to health improvement...to prolong and multiply health gains many times over.[2]

---

2 Hawe, P., Noort, M., King, L., Jorden, C. (1997), 'Multiplying Health Gains: the Critical Role of Capacity Building in Health Promotion Programs', *Health Policy*, 39, pp. 29–42.

It is sometimes described as the invisible work of health promotion. It has been described as including activities as diverse as canvassing the opportunities for a program, lobbying for support, developing skills, supporting policy development, negotiating with management, partnerships development and organisational planning.

Commentary

The model developed by Goodman and colleagues is particularly helpful in illustrating the ways in which organisations function at different levels, how the achievement of organisational change may be achieved in a staged process, and how each stage may require involvement of different levels in an organisation. The model is most useful in situations where an organisation is viewed as a potential host institution to previously developed health programs. It does not so easily accommodate health promotion strategies that seek to help organisations to develop in a more holistic way, such as to develop organisational policy and practices, as a means to creating safe and health-supportive environments for workers and clients.

Models of intersectoral action

As well as working with organisations as potential host institutions for existing programs, and as a means to creating supportive environments for health, we need increasingly to work with organisations as partners in the development and implementation of health promotion programs. This process is often referred to as intersectoral action. The World Health Organization (WHO) defines intersectoral action for health as:

> a recognised relationship between part or parts of the health sector with part or parts of other sectors which has been formed to take action on an issue to achieve a health outcome…in a way that is more effective, efficient or sustainable than could be achieved by the health sector working alone.

There are few theories or models that define this process and none that enjoy universal recognition among health promotion workers, but there have been several recent attempts to review experience in intersectoral action and in related activities such as coalition-building and partnerships. These reviews have identified different forms of intersectoral action and sets of factors that are important to understanding the process by which organisations, or parts of organisations, work together.

Glendinning and colleagues have identified that two of the most fundamental factors that influence the nature and success of intersectoral working are the extent of dependence and the trust between partner organisations. Put simply, if one organisation depends upon cooperation with another to achieve their goals, and there exists a high level of trust between them, then joint action is more feasible and more likely to be successful. By working together organisations may be able to ensure that their services are more relevant and coordinated, and have access to sufficient resources to make a difference. For example, food suppliers and distributors may be willing to work with the health sector to improve the supply of fresh fruit and vegetables to an area. The food suppliers would do so with the intention of increasing sales of these foods (their core business). The health sector will do so to improve nutrition in a population (their core business). The partners are to some extent codependent, each able to achieve their core business more successfully by working together than by working in isolation.

Trust between organisations is also crucial to the development of strong intersectoral partnerships. Trust is developed over time and is built on relationships between individuals and their organisations. For this reason many successful partnerships are between individuals and organisations that have worked successfully together in the past. The relationships that develop are based on respect for all those involved and recognition of their unique capacity to contribute to achieving their shared goals. Building trust can be very challenging. In many relationships between organisations there is an imbalance in control over resources and capacity to influence decision-making. There may also have been a history of competition or antagonism between the organisations. In these cases it becomes essential that the relationship and the benefits to all those involved is transparent and fair.

Although we often speak of partnerships or coalitions, it is important to remember that there is no one model of the way in which organisations work together. At one end of the spectrum, the relationships between organisations may be simply one of sharing information and meeting regularly to discuss common problems. At the other end of the spectrum, partnerships can be highly structured, where the roles, responsibilities and outcomes are mandated.

Figure 5.1 identifies a continuum between networks, alliances, partnerships, coalitions and highly structured collaborations developed by O'Neill and colleagues. This continuum reflects increased formal agreements between organisations to work

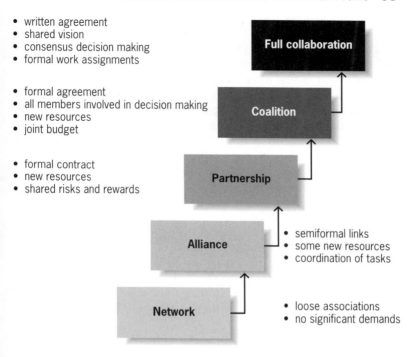

- written agreement
- shared vision
- consensus decision making
- formal work assignments

Full collaboration

- formal agreement
- all members involved in decision making
- new resources
- joint budget

Coalition

- formal contract
- new resources
- shared risks and rewards

Partnership

Alliance

- semiformal links
- some new resources
- coordination of tasks

Network

- loose associations
- no significant demands

Figure 5.1 Continuum of ways organisations work together

together in certain areas and a greater investment of organisational resources.

Beyond these basic factors of codependence and trust, a review of intersectoral action in Australia has proposed a framework for understanding the factors that will influence effective intersectoral action. In this model six factors were identified as important dimensions to effective intersectoral action:

1. the necessity for the sectors or organisations to work together;
2. the factors that are providing the opportunity for them to work together;
3. the capacity to work together;
4. established relationships that will allow them to achieve their goal;
5. the action they are undertaking should be planned and able to be evaluated; and
6. the action should be sustainable.

Understanding the context

Successful collaboration between organisations needs to build on the foundations of necessity and opportunity. Organisations are more likely to be open to collaboration and change if it helps them to pursue core business more effectively or efficiently. This core business may have nothing to do with health in a direct sense, but may have an indirect impact on health, for example, if the core business is transport or housing programs, or the activities of private sector companies promoting different foods. In addition to achieving their organisational goals, organisations are also interested in working together to:

- attract or protect resources;
- protect or gain in their areas of influence; and
- be seen as good corporate citizens.

Understanding the strength of the motivation for organisations to work together assists in understanding the level of commitment they will be willing to make, and of the risk they will be willing to take.

> Successful collaboration between organisations needs to build on the foundations of necessity and opportunity.

The opportunity for taking action is reflected in immediate organisational priorities. These may be in response to crises within organisations, or a response to unpredicted events outside the organisation, for example, a number of fatal football injuries may make it more likely that sporting organisations will be receptive to advice concerning changes in rules recommended by the health sector. However, without the infrastructure to undertake action, such opportunities to work with other organisations to achieve common goals may be missed.

Assessing the infrastructure

Many of the factors which contribute to either the success or the failure of a particular activity are seen as related to the capacity of the organisations to undertake that activity. This capacity is primarily reflected in:

- the level of organisational support for the activity (including compatible structures and decision-making processes);
- adequate levels of resources (including time, financial resources and infrastructure); and
- a skilled workforce.

The other crucial aspect of infrastructure is the relationship that exists between the organisations involved. These relationships are generally a mix of formal and informal links, and provide the mechanism within which actions can be developed and conflicts resolved.

Without adequate infrastructure it can be difficult for organisations to sustain action over time or adapt to changing circumstances.

A planned approach to action and sustainability

Building and sustaining relationships between sectors towards common goals is a difficult task. Many of the conditions for success (or failure) are in place long before any specific action is taken and it is important not only to plan the details of the project, but also to account for the context in which it is being undertaken and the ability of the infrastructure of the organisations to deliver. From reviews of practice, several issues have emerged as important in the implementation of a project that requires cooperation between different agencies:

- clear recognition of why it is important for the organisations to work together, including agreement on how the issue and the solution are defined, and what role they see for their respective organisations in the implementation process;
- acknowledgment that the process is emergent and changing;
- the need for flexibility in negotiation over roles and responsibilities;
- definition of a clearly articulated and achievable goal that is understood and valued by the different organisations involved in a project;
- agreement on a way of working—this may mean working on small, well-defined tasks initially to build trust and confidence in a working relationship before seeking to implement more significant changes;
- opportunities for renegotiation including identification of the length of time to which organisations are committed, and allowing for redefinition of tasks, roles and relationships;

- commitment to joint ownership—any sense that one partner is imposing on another invariably leads to resistance and damage to the relationship; and
- allocation of resources—staff, space, money, information and administrative support.

Commentary

As many of the most entrenched health problems we face, especially those related to addressing health inequality, have their roots in the wider social system it is inevitable that health promotion workers will continue to need to work across organisations to improve health. For these reasons, the concepts and values that underpin notions of collaboration and partnership have resonance with many health promotion workers. They sit easily with a recognition that action to improve health is not only the responsibility of the health system, but also that of many other organisations. This has led to a high level of investment in partnership working, coalition building and the types of intersectoral action described above.

However, there is increasing concern that the level of investment that is required in establishing and maintaining effective relationships may be greater than the benefits. For this reason it is important to develop a critical approach to deciding if, and how, these relationships should be developed and what it is that we hope will be achieved by them.

Although there is not a single agreed model or theory of intersectoral action there is now a strong body of experience that provides some guidance on those factors that are important in effective action. There is also a better understanding that the relationships between organisations can take many forms and that it is not always essential to establish highly formalised relationships if the organisational goals of all those involved can be met through more informal means.

It is also clear that if organisations are to work effectively together they often need to change internally in order for them to have the capacity to work with other organisations: for example, they may need to change their funding cycle or processes for making decisions. In particular they may need to employ staff who are able to work effectively across organisations.

Summary

Although the models described above are not strictly theories according to the criteria described at the beginning of the book, they are based on systematic observation and analysis of organisational change, and do offer guidance on factors influencing the successful introduction and maintenance of change in organisational settings. Further, systematic testing of these ideas in planned programs will be necessary to clarify their usefulness and identify further refinements.

These models provide useful guidance on the different steps required to introduce and sustain a program in different organisational settings. In particular they highlight:

- the need to understand the core business of an organisation and its organisational structure, and determine how a health promotion program can fit within these parameters, and help achieve core business;
- the need to work with individuals at different levels in an organisation as well as between organisations;
- the inherently 'political' nature of the task of influencing senior managers;
- the importance of flexibility in negotiation with 'gatekeepers' concerning the adoption of a program;
- the need to support those individuals responsible for the delivery of a program or innovation; and
- the need to establish a system for long-term maintenance and quality control.

One of the major reasons that the health sector is interested in working with other organisational structures is to bring about systematic and lasting change that will address some of the basic determinants of health, for example, safe workplaces, improved living conditions or the development of recreational facilities. Understanding how to do this most effectively has the potential to have profound impacts on health.

Further reading

Theories of organisational change

Goodman, R.M., Steckler, A., Kegler, M.C. (2002), 'Mobilizing Organizations for Health Enhancement: Theories of Organizational Change', in Glanz, K. et al. *Health Behavior and Health Education: Theory, Research and Practice*, 3rd edition, Jossey-Bass, San Francisco, California.

Hawe, P., Noort, M., King, L., Jorden, C. (1997), 'Multiplying Health Gains: the Critical Role of Capacity Building in Health Promotion Programs', *Health Policy*, 39, pp. 29–42.

Models of intersectoral action

Butterfoss, F.D., Goodman, R., Wandersman, A. (1993), 'Community Coalitions for Prevention and Health Promotion', *Health Education Research*, 8, 3, pp. 315–330.

Glendinning, C., Powell, M., Rummery, K. (eds) (2002), *Partnerships, New Labour and the Governance of Welfare*, Policy Press, Bristol.

Harris, E., Wise, M., Hawe, P. et al. (1995), *Working Together: Intersectoral Action for Health*, Australian Government Publishing Service, Canberra.

O'Neill, M., Lemieux, V., Groleau, G. et al. (1997), 'Coalition theory as a framework for understanding and implementing intersectoral health-related interventions', *Health Promotion International*, 12, 1, pp. 79–85.

World Health Organization International Conference on Intersectoral Action for Health (1997), Geneva.

Chapter 6
Models for the development of healthy public policy

he mounting evidence that factors outside the control of the health sector have a profound impact on health has resulted in increasing interest in the development of public policies that protect and promote health. For example, housing, income support, employment, education, and environmental protection policies can have both a direct and an indirect impact on the health of individuals and communities.

How can the policies that impact on health be influenced? This is still a developing area of study in health promotion. This section examines three frameworks that have been proposed by people working in the area of health promotion for understanding the development of healthy public policy.

A framework for making healthy public policy

Nancy Milio has proposed a conceptual framework through which we can develop a greater appreciation of how successful public policy to improve health is developed.

In this framework, policy development is seen as passing through discrete stages of initiation, adoption, implementation, evaluation and reformulation. These stages are part of a continuous social and political process that is not strictly linear. The development of healthy public policy is seen as a dynamic process and not simply the production of a policy statement.

In this framework there are four main players who are crucial in the development of healthy public policy:

1. policy makers (usually politicians and bureaucracies);

2. policy influencers (who can be groups inside and outside of government);
3. the public (audiences, consumers, taxpayers and voters) whose opinion will ultimately affect the adoption of the policy; and
4. the media (print and electronic) that influence both the policy makers' and the public's understanding of, and attitude towards, an issue.

Although the development of healthy public policy often appears to be driven by one or a group of influential individuals, Milio argues that it is the organisations and not the individuals that lead them that should be the focus of analysis. This gives a better understanding of the motivation and resource base of those involved.

> The development of healthy public policy is seen as a dynamic process and not simply the production of a policy statement.

Within organisations the key stakeholders are seen as falling broadly into two groups: the policy makers who have initiated or hold a mandate for a specific policy and move the policy at a pace based on their interests; and the policy influencers who have an interest in the issue and may try to influence the content of the policy and the speed and way in which it is implemented. For example, the police may be seen as the policy keepers in gun regulation while the policy influencers may consist of gun lobbies, public health bodies and community coalitions.

In this model the general public is not seen as influencing the formulation of specific policies in important ways, but is seen as forming part of the climate for policy making.

A number of key determinants of influencing policy development are identified:

- the social, economic and political context in which action is proposed (social climate);
- the identification of parties with most influence on policy development;
- the recognition of the interests of those wishing to influence policy development (what they will win or lose, where they are willing to compromise); and

- the capacity of those wishing to develop or influence policy to put in place strategies that will be successful in representing their interests.

The social climate in which the policy is being developed has a significant impact on the relatively few political leaders who will finally make the decision to adopt a policy. For example, in the gun control debate in Australia a number of tragic mass shootings dramatically shifted the social climate from a concern for the rights of shooters towards the broader community interest to be protected from the consequences of uncontrolled access to guns.

In this case the groups wanting tighter gun control found that their power to influence change had increased. They were better placed to put forward tough proposals for gun control in the belief that government would be unlikely to ignore broad-based support. Those groups against gun control needed to find ways to re-exert their influence and put forward arguments to the government that would counterbalance community sentiments.

Milio argues that how major stakeholders respond will be coloured by what they see as in their best long-term interests. This may differ from their public statements. Groups may choose not to influence the development of the policy but rather put their effort into opposing the implementation of the policy.

Finally, it is important to understand that major players, both within and outside government, will develop strategic plans to influence the development of policies that have a high priority. The type and effectiveness of this strategy will depend on such things as the size of the organisation, their resources, organisational age (affecting experience, contacts and credibility), their authority (closeness and importance to the policy makers), and their skill in using these assets.

Developing effective information strategies will be an important part of this process. For example, in the gun debate, having credible spokespersons who could provide leadership and information was an important factor in developing a climate that would support change. Milio argues that the ways in which information is used will vary. It can be less active use of information to monitor, analyse and critique policy making; or more direct efforts in persuading, mediating or mobilising others to action. This can be directed at the policy makers themselves or past them to influence credible public figures to support the issue and/or build public support. Milio sees that the media has a central role in creating public opinion not only by what they report but also by choosing whether to say anything at all, who is allowed to speak, how much prominence an issue is given and the way the issue is framed. The role of the media becomes very important when this information is not available to policy makers or the public through experience or other sources.

Commentary

This model presents a clear picture of the groups who have a role in policy development—the policy makers, interested parties, the public and the media. It highlights the need to see policy development as a dynamic process that can be influenced at many stages by those who have something to win or lose, and by the social climate in which the policy makers are operating. How this social climate is shaped will depend very much on how the media report, or fail to report, the issue.

Evidence-based policy making to promote health

> Evidence will be used in a variety of ways to lead, justify or support policy development.

Even the most casual observer of healthy public policy can see that there is often a poor relationship between what is known about factors that cause or could prevent illness and disability and the policies in place about these issues. As the range and quality of research and evaluation on health promotion has grown, so too has the case for 'evidence-based' policy making for health. Epidemiologists and other population health researchers often complain that their findings are not taken up by policy makers, while policy makers complain that there is often no relevant evidence for them to base policy on. Neither position is completely accurate.

In reality, evidence will be used in a variety of ways to lead, justify or support policy development. The examination of the relationship between evidence and policy is not new. Carol Weiss is generally considered to be among the pioneers of the study of this relationship and has developed a set of models which help explain the different ways in which evidence has been used to guide the policy making process. These include:

- **The knowledge-driven model.** In this model the emergence of new knowledge from research will automatically create pressure for its application in policy. In such a model, there is a relatively quick transfer of new knowledge into policy development. In public health, the development of new vaccines will often lead to public pressure for their immediate adoption, even when an analysis of benefit relative to cost indicates that there may be alternative investments that could produce greater public health improvements.

- **The problem-solving model.** In this model, evidence derived from a variety of sources is gathered and applied as a starting point for the development of policy. This problem-solving model implies that mechanisms exist in policy making to gather and apply evidence as the primary driver of decision making in the development of policy. It suggests that policy making is a rational, iterative process with a clear beginning and end.

- **The interactive model.** Here, research knowledge is utilised as one input in the decision-making process, alongside experience, political insight and social pressures. This corresponds more closely to the description of the policy-making process described by Milio in the previous section.

- **The political model.** In this model, evidence is used to justify a predetermined position. It reflects a more overtly 'political' use of evidence, and commonly relies upon a selective inclusion of favourable data, and the interpretation of facts and events to fit with predetermined positions. The exclusive use of mass media campaigns and of school-based interventions to address complex problems, such as drug misuse and antisocial behaviour, can be seen as examples of this model.

- **The tactical model.** Here, evidence is used to delay a decision or to avoid responsibility for an unpopular decision. In this model the normal uncertainty of research findings is exploited as a mechanism for delaying a decision until 'more evidence is gathered'. Alternatively, where an unpopular decision is made, evidence may be used to justify that decision, even if the evidence is rather weak.

Weiss' work is helpful in illustrating the range of ways in which evidence is used to support the policy-making process. Although it is comforting to believe that there is a seamless and rational relationship between the development of knowledge and its application to policy (as implied in the knowledge-driven and problem-solving models), in reality there is rarely such a simple relationship between research and policy. The work of Nancy Milio and Weiss suggests that it is more likely that evidence will be used in policy development in ways that correspond to the interactive, political and tactical models described above.

It follows that policy making is rarely an 'event', or even an explicit set of decisions derived from an appraisal of evidence and following a preplanned course. Policy tends to evolve through an iterative process, subject to continuous review and incremental change. Policy making is an inherently 'political' process, and the timing of decisions is usually dictated as much by political considerations as by the state of the evidence. As such policy making requires a point in time appraisal of:

- what is scientifically plausible (evidence based);
- what is politically acceptable (fit with political vision); and
- what is practical for implementation.

  In this context, policy is most likely to be evidence based if:

- evidence is available and accessible at the time it is needed;
- the evidence fits with political vision (or can be made to fit); and
- the evidence points to actions for which powers and resources are (or could be) available, and the systems, structures and capacity for action exist.

Scientists frequently complain that their research is ignored by policy makers. Weiss' work makes clear that this may well be true, by fault or by design. However, researchers also need to examine the extent to which their choice of subject, methods of communication, and lack of understanding of the policy process contribute to the fact that their important work is ignored.

Evelyn De Leeuw has proposed that there are three determinants of policy making that need to be understood if those interested in the development of healthy public policy are to make progress:

1. the bias that stems from sets of causal, final and normative assumptions and presuppositions;
2. the interest webs of groups in certain domains; and
3. the power of organisations to monitor and communicate their intentions.

Assumptions

Policy makers acquire in their career and work environment a set of assumptions and beliefs about general policy directions. Three sets of assumptions that affect policy development are proposed: those around the relationship between cause and effect; those between intervention and outcome; and underlying values. Together they are seen as forming a set of assumptions and presuppositions that is the framework in which policy objectives, instruments and time frames are established and assessed. Very rarely are these assumptions and presuppositions made explicit, although they set the parameters of action that will be seen as desirable and feasible.

For example, in exerting pressure for the development of policies to address the health impact of unemployment, these three sets of assumptions appear to influence the views of those involved. The relationship between unemployment (cause) and poor health (effect) is often perceived to be unclear—were the unemployed more likely to have lost their job because they were sick, or is their poor health due to an unhealthy lifestyle rather than unemployment itself? There may be simplistic views about the nature of the interventions that may bring about changes in health outcomes, for instance that full employment will solve the problem. And despite the fact that there are far fewer jobs available than people to fill them, there still seem to be views in the community that people could find a job if they really wanted to work, as reflected in keeping job-seeking diaries etc.

Interests

The way policy is formulated and implemented is often determined by the vested interests of stakeholders or interest groups. For example, in efforts to reduce unemployment levels there are many vested interests that can range from those trying to deregulate the labour market as a way of promoting economic growth, through to unions who may be interested in seeing that their members do not lose their jobs, and to welfare groups advocating better income support for people who are unemployed.

As well as wanting to see a reduction in unemployment, these groups need to ensure their own survival and spheres of influence. De Leeuw argues that they are often willing to undertake any action to ensure their survival. If action is to be taken that will protect and promote health then those developing the policies need to recognise the different and overlapping areas of interest and perceived needs.

Providing health-based information by itself may not meet this need.

> The way policy is formulated and implemented is often determined by the vested interests of stakeholders or interest groups.

Power positions

The effectiveness that groups will have in exerting their power or influence is seen as closely related to their capacity to understand the policy and strategic intentions of their competitors and allies. For example, if the health sector is trying to introduce policies to reduce the impact of unemployment on health it needs to recognise that less powerful interest groups may see the health sector's interest as being a way to get more money for services or as cost shifting.

The perceived power of those involved affects any strategic action taken. The degree of power that groups have, their capacity to monitor the interests and plans of others, and their ability to communicate their own intentions has proved highly predictive in the success organisations have in influencing policy.

De Leeuw's focus is on how epidemiological information can inform policy development to promote health. It is not enough to know or even communicate the 'truth'; attempts also need to be made to use this information in ways that will be taken up by major stakeholders. This involves understanding how they see the issue, how they think it is caused, how they think action will be effective, the nature of the stakeholders' interests and the way in which health interests may potentially benefit them, and a detailed understanding of the strategies used by those involved to achieve their organisational ends.

Commentary

The models proposed by Weiss helpfully describe the ways in which research can inform and direct the development of public policy for health, but do not offer clear advice on how practitioners can better influence events. Observations on the need to consider timing, presentation and practical application of research findings complement Weiss' work. The model developed by De Leeuw to understand the factors that will influence the development of healthy public policy provides a way of understanding why many attempts to promote a particular policy fail. It is not only because of the power of the groups involved or what they stand to gain or lose. Willingness to support a particular issue will also be influenced by what those involved believe to be the cause of the problem, what they feel can effectively be done to address it, and their assumptions and presuppositions about where health is created. De Leeuw's work is derived from and linked back to the model proposed by Milio in the previous section.

Impact assessment and health impact assessment

In recent years there has been an increasing focus on different types of 'impact assessment' and ways that they can contribute to policy development and implementation. In the public health context this has focused particularly on the development of 'health impact assessment' (HIA). As its name suggests this essentially involves assessing potential impacts of a particular proposal on the health of a defined population. This ability to consider and assess the potential impact of policy and service developments on defined populations (e.g. in a geographical area, or a specific social group) is increasingly becoming a core competency for health promotion practitioners who wish to inform and influence the decision-making process.

Currently there is a range of different types of impact assessment that provide models for adaptation to HIA. These include environmental, economic and regulatory impact assessments. Some forms of assessment are mandatory in different countries, mostly to determine the likely economic impact and/or impact on quality of life for populations affected by policy change. Slowly, requirements for HIA are emerging. For example, in the European Union (EU), the Amsterdam Treaty (Article 152) calls for the EU to examine major policies for their potential impact on health.

As different types of impact assessment have developed so too has work to find ways to achieve better connection and integration between them.

Informing decision making

It is possible to consider HIA in a range of ways. In some respects it represents common sense as much as a particular process using a set of individual methods and approaches. It is clearly possible to look at any policy or practice and consider its potential impact on a specific issue. Most policy makers and practitioners would probably argue that they are involved in doing this on a routine basis. However, where undertaking a dedicated HIA can be of particular value is in helping ensure that the assumptions and decisions that underlie the development of a policy or practice are made transparent and open to wider consideration and discussion by those that are affected.

HIA has the potential to inform and open up decision-making processes by clarifying underlying assumptions and ensuring the evidence of potential impacts is considered. If undertaken well it can do this in a way that can be reviewed and tested over time, thereby not only helping to directly inform particular decisions but also having the potential to contribute to a growing evidence base for effective policy and practice over time.

A flexible and adaptable approach

As a potential tool to inform decision making, HIA is flexible and adaptable. It can incorporate a range of approaches and methods with no single methodology or 'right way' to do it. To date this has proved both an advantage, in helping ensure it can be specifically tailored to individual circumstances and requirements as resources allow, and also a problem in that it can lead to variations in the quality and utility of the assessments.

The time needed to undertake a HIA can vary from a matter of days to many months depending on the available time and resources to inform the decision-making process. Nevertheless, whatever time is available there is increasing consensus on the major stages that are core to any HIA process. These are described below.

Screening: deciding whether to undertake a HIA

As a HIA is only one way to inform decision making it is important to consider and rule out the utility of other potential approaches before deciding to proceed. A major consideration here is making a judgement of the extent any HIA is likely to be valued by the relevant decision makers. The primary purpose of HIA is to inform particular decisions. However good, it will be of little value if the relevant decision makers are not engaged and open to considering its recommendations. If there is reluctance to wait for an assessment, or resistance to potential findings, health promotion practitioners need to consider alternative routes to influence policy.

Scoping: deciding how to undertake the HIA in the available time

Once it has been decided to undertake a HIA it is necessary to examine the best way to do this given the available time and resources. The central consideration, whatever process is adopted, is ensuring that it can be completed in time to generate clear recommendations for the relevant decision makers and in enough time to be considered ahead of any decisions being made. This is one of the most difficult challenges for this methodology, as it often takes too long to execute to meet political deadlines. The methodology has to be adapted to meet the time available.

Appraisal: identifying and examining evidence for potential impacts

This is the core stage of the HIA process and essentially involves:

- identifying potential ways that a proposal might be expected to have an impact on the health of a population (both positively and negatively); and
- examining what different types of evidence can support a judgement about the potential significance and scale of such impacts.

Issues of particular importance at this stage include:

- Systematically examining the ways a proposal may affect major underlying influences on health including socioeconomic factors; environmental conditions; social, community and working contexts; individual and family lifestyles.
- Considering disproportionate impacts on populations—it may have potential equity or health inequality impacts.
- Examining different stakeholder perspectives on a proposal to assess potential impacts. When done well the HIA process can have value in supporting stakeholder engagement with both communities who will be directly affected and key decision makers.
- Incorporating and valuing different sources of evidence. Assessing evidence for impacts in complex and dynamic social systems presents a range of challenges. Evidence drawn from a mix of different disciplines, from physical sciences and biomedicine to broader psychological and sociological approaches, is important.

Producing recommendations: deciding on what to recommend to the relevant decision makers

Key to this stage is understanding the values and requirements of the relevant decision makers, so that a set of recommendations can be developed which are likely to be seriously considered and valued by them, and thereby have the greatest chance of being adopted. Crucial to framing such recommendations will be a recognition that decision makers are likely to be considering a range of factors, with health probably only one of them. Helping link the potential health benefits to other considerations, such as economic issues, employment, education, housing and regeneration, is likely to enhance the HIA's perceived value.

Review and evaluation

Once the recommendations have been produced and considered by the decision makers the purpose of the HIA is essentially complete. However, routine review and evaluation of the contribution of the assessment should be seen as a fundamental part of planning and undertaking a good process.

In particular such review needs to address the extent to which:

- the HIA's recommendations were actually adopted by the relevant decision makers, and the reason why all, or some, were adopted;
- adopted recommendations had the predicted positive impacts;
- not adopted recommendations had the predicated negative impacts; and
- there were other unanticipated positive or negative impacts arising from the proposal.

Commentary

HIA is an emerging tool that has great potential to influence the policy-making process. Its strength is in the extent to which it offers a systematic approach to the examination of policy development. At best, it opens up decision-making processes, by clarifying underlying assumptions and ensuring that the best available evidence can inform them. It also offers considerable scope to provide a voice to those individuals and communities most affected by the emerging policy. The major problems encountered by proponents of HIA are the extent to which it is recognised as a legitimate tool in the policy-making process (for example, in comparison to environmental or regulatory impact assessments) and the time taken to complete the process. In the former case, the methodology is not yet sufficiently established, nor has it been considered sufficiently robust, to warrant serious attention by many policy makers. In the latter case, information derived from HIA runs the risk of being produced too late to be of significant influence on the decision-making process. Greater use of HIA, and further development of more flexible and responsive methodologies, will do much to overcome some of these deficits.

Summary

Taken together these three approaches provide us with valuable guidance on how healthy public policy can be developed and influenced by researchers and practitioners, as well as providing guidance in assessing the impact of policies on health.

They stress the need to recognise that policy is not based solely on the evidence of the nature and extent of the problem and what are thought by health promotion practitioners to be effective strategies to address it.

In order to understand the process through which policy is developed it is important to recognise the major stakeholders and their interests, recognise their perceptions of the issue and their possible solutions, and understand possible areas of conflict and compromise.

Although not directly influential in policy development, the importance of public opinion and the general climate in which the organisations are operating are also highlighted as important. Influencing these opinions and environments is recognised as important in introducing new ideas and having policies adopted.

Further reading

A framework for making healthy public policy

Milio, N. (1987), 'Making healthy public policy: developing the science by learning the art: an ecological framework for policy studies', *Health Promotion*, 2, 3, pp. 263–274.

Evidence-based policy making to promote health

De Leeuw, E. (1993), 'Health policy, epidemiology and power: the interest web', *Health Promotion International*, 8, 1, pp. 49–53.

Nutbeam, D. (2001), 'Evidence-based public policy for health: matching research to policy need', *Promotion and Education*, 2, pp. 15–19.

Weiss, C.H. (1979), 'The Many Meanings of Research Utilisation', *Public Administration Review*, 39, pp. 426–431.

Further web-based sources of information on HIA

The World Health Organization: http://www.who.int/hia

A dedicated HIA website resource is maintained by the Health Development Agency: www.hiagateway.org.uk

The European Centre for Health Policy has useful web pages on HIA: www.who.dk/hs/ECHP/index.htm

The International Association of Impact Assessment has a dedicated HIA section: www.iaia.org

Conclusion
Theory in practice

This book provides only an introduction to the many different theories and models that have guided health promotion practice. In each case the different chapters provide a synthesis of the different elements of the theories and the research that has guided their development, and indicate their reliability for guidance of practice. Readers who require more detailed information on the different theories should refer to the original texts cited at the end of each chapter, or to other more comprehensive publications.

What will be apparent from the different chapters is that the theory guiding practice in health promotion is not yet well developed. The theories concerning psychosocial determinants of health in individuals are the least complex and best tested according to traditional criteria. The different theories and models that may be useful to guide elements of programs directed to community mobilisation, organisational change and policy development are generally less well formed and far less amenable to testing through typical experimental research designs such as randomised controlled trials. In such cases these models may represent part of the art of health promotion as much as they represent the science. However, the importance of community mobilisation and organisational and policy change for health is so great that it is essential to identify and apply our best current understanding of these issues. Research to advance our knowledge and understanding of such processes is of the highest priority in the future.

There is no single theory or model that can adequately guide the development of a comprehensive health promotion program intended to influence the multiple determinants of health in populations. Practitioners need to use local knowledge and experience, and available research information to make judgments about community needs and the determinants of health that are most amenable to change at any particular time. In developing a comprehensive strategy to tackle a defined health priority, practitioners will be assisted by making judicious use of the theories and models described in this book. Multilevel interventions will generally be more powerful than single-track programs. Correspondingly, programs will need to draw on several of the theories and models described in this book in the development of a comprehensive strategy. If applied wisely, these theories will help guide decisions, may predict the likely outcomes and help explain the reasons for success.

Not all practitioners have the position or capacity to operate at multiple levels. In such cases knowledge of the theories in this book will help practitioners to maximise the potential effectiveness of their interventions, and to place into perspective their efforts alongside the range of opportunities for action.

Index

Page numbers in **bold** print refer to main entries

access (health program), 13, 45
action models, intersectorial, xii, xiii, 4, **53–8**
action stage (change), 17, 18
addictive behaviours, 17
adopter classification (Rogers), 26, **27–8**
adoption process (innovation), 28–9
adoption stage (organisational change), **51**
AIDS campaign, 12, 13
Ajzen, I., 14, 15, 16
alliances, 54, 55
Amsterdam Treaty, 69
appraisal (HIA), **71**
assumptions, 66, **67**, 70
attention, 41
attitudes, 14, 15, 39, 40, **41**, 42
awareness raising, xi, 3, 4, 6, 41
awareness raising stage (organisational change), **50–1**

Bandura, Albert, 19, 20, 21, 30
barriers see perceived barriers
behavioural beliefs, 14
behavioural capacity, 21
behavioural intentions, 14, 15
beliefs, xi, xiii, 2, 6, **10–14**, 15, 16, 21, 22, 23, 39, 40, 42, 67
bias, 66
Bush, R., 33, 34

capacity, community, 31, **33–4**, **35**, 36
capacity, organisational, **52–3**, 56–7
capacity building, 4, 32, 51, **52–3**
change agents, 22, 27, 29, 37
change maintenance, 41, 51
channel of communication, **40**, 41, 45, 46
characteristics (personal), 2, 11, 21
climate see organisational climate
coalition building, 53, 54, 55, 58
collaboration, 54, 55, **56**, 58
collective perception, 52
commercial marketing, 43, 44
communication–behaviour change model, xi, xiii, 4, **39–42**, 45, 46
communication channels, **40**, 41, 45, 46
    see also mass communication
communication inputs, **39–40**
communication outputs, **41**
community, theories on change in, **25–30**
community building and community organisation, xi, xiii, 25, **30–6**
community capacity, 31, **33–4**, **35**, 36
community competence, xi
community development, 32
community empowerment, 32, 33, 35, 36, 37
community health promotion, 7

community interest, 63
community mobilisation, 31, 75
community organisation and
    community building, xi, xiii,
    25, **30–6**
consciousness raising, 18
contemplation stage (change),
    17, 18
control beliefs, 14
core business, 56, 59
corporate citizenship, 56
cost effectiveness, 29
cues, 22
cultural values, 29
culture *see* organisational culture

De Leeuw, Evelyn, 66, 67, 68–9
decision making, informing, **69–70**
'decisional balance', 17
demographic variables, 40
dependence, **54**, 55
destination (communication), 40
determination stage (change),
    17, 18
DiClimente, C.C., 16
diffusion defined, 26
diffusion of innovation theory, xi,
    4, 25, **26–30**, 36, 50
direct selling, 45
Dower, J., 33, 34

early adopters, 27, 28
early majority, 27, 28
education, health, 12, 13, 23,
    39, 42
empowerment, 32, 33, 35, 36, 37
empowerment 'continuum', **32–3**
environmental influences, 4, **20**,
    22, 23, 52
    see also social environment
evaluation stages
    health impact assessment, **72**
    health promotion program, 2,
        3, **5–6**
    use of theory in, 2, 3, **5–6**, 7
evidence-based policy making,
    xii, xiii, **64–9**
expectations
    health belief model, 11
    social cognitive theory, 21

experience, 4
exposure, 41

Fishbein, M., 14, 15, 16
four Ps, **44–5**, 46–7

gatekeepers, 51, 59
general practitioners and the
    transtheoretical model, **17–18**
Glanz, Karen, 8
Glendinning, C., 54
goals *see* organisational goals
Goodman, R.M., 33, 49, 50, 52, 53
Green, W.W., 2
gun control debate, 63

Hawe, P., 52
health behaviour and health
    behaviour change theories,
    10–24
health belief model, xi, xiii, 2, 5,
    10–14, 46
health care service/resource
    access, 13
health education, 12, 13, 23,
    39, 42
health impact assessment, xiii,
    69–73
health inequality, 58
health messages, xi–xii, 40, 41, 45,
    46, 47
health outcome assessment, 5
health promotion, xi–xii, xiii, 1,
    22, 30
health promotion interventions,
    16, 20
health promotion outcomes, 5
health promotion planning and
    evaluation cycle, 2, **3–4**
health promotion programs, 23,
    46–7
health screening services, 45
health-supportive organisational
    practice, **49–60**
healthy public policy
    evidence-based, xii, xiii, **64–9**
    framework for making, xii, xiii,
        61–4
    impact assessment and health
        impact, xii, xiii, **69–73**

models for development of,
61–74
HIA, xiii, **69–73**
HIV infection, **11–12**, 13, 16

immunisation programs, 7, 43, 45
impact assessment, xii, xiii, 3, 5,
6, **69–73**
implementation stage
health promotion program, 2,
3, **4**, **5**, **6**
mobilising resources for, **4**, 6
organisational change, **51**
individual health promotion, 7
information technology, 40
informing decision making (HIA),
69–70
infrastructure assessment, 34,
56–7
innovation defined, 26
innovation diffusion, xi, xiii, 4,
25, **26–30**, 36, 50
innovation maintenance, 51
innovators, 27, 28
institutionalisation stage
(organisational change), **51**
interactive model (evidence-based
policy making), **65**
interest webs, 66
interests (evidence-based policy
making), **67–8**
intermediate outcome
assessment, 5
intersectorial action models, xii,
xiii, 4, **53–8**
intervention, multilevel, 76
intervention combinations, 7
intervention focus, 2
intervention methods, 46
intervention targets, 3
intervention theories, **7**, 8
intervention timing and
sequencing, 4

joint ownership, 58

knowledge, 39
knowledge-driven model, **65**, 66
knowledge transfer, 33
Kreuter, M.W., 2

laggards, 27, 28, 30
late majority, 27, 28
learning
observational, 20, 21
participatory, 21
lobbying, 53
locality development, **31**, 32

Maibach, E.W., 42
maintenance (change), 41, 51
maintenance stage
(transtheoretical model),
17, 18
market research, 44, 47
marketing, **43**
marketing analysis, **44**
marketing mix, **44–5**
marketing organisations, 42–3
mass communication, xi, 37, 40,
46, **47**
mass media, 42, 65
McGuire, W.J., 39–40, 45
media, 4, 11, 40–1, 42, 45, 47, 62,
63–4, 65
memorisation, 41
message, xi–xii, 40, 41, 45, 46, 47
Milio, Nancy, 61, 62, 63–4, 66, 69
Minkler, M., 32
mobilisation, community, 31, 75
motivation
social cognitive theory and, 21
theory of reasoned action
and, 14
multilevel interventions, 76
Mutch, A., 33

network partnerships, 33
networks, 54, 55
normative beliefs, 14
norms *see* organisational norms;
social norms; subjective
norms
Novelli, W.D., 44

observation, 4, 23
observational learning, 20, 21
O'Neill, M., 54
opportunity costs, 45
organisational capacity, **52–3**,
56–7

organisational change theory, xii, xiii, 3, 4, **49–53**, 59
organisational climate, **52**, 63
organisational culture, **52**
organisational development, 6
organisational goals, 56, 58
organisational health promotion, 7
organisational norms, 52
organisational policy, 4
organisational practices, 4, 6, 7
organisational priorities, 56
organisational procedures, 4
organisational relationships, 57
organisational structures, xii, 1, 49, 59
organisational values, 52
Ottawa Charter for Health Promotion, 7
outcome expectations, 11, 21

participatory learning, 21
partnerships, 4, 6, 53, **54**, 55, 58
peer pressure/influences, 15, 16, 20, 23
perceived barriers, 11, 12, 13, 15, 17
perceived behavioural control, 15
perceived benefits, 11, 12, 13
perceived power, 14, 15, 68
perceived seriousness, 10, 11
perceived susceptibility, 10, 11, 12
perceived threat, 11
personal characteristics, 2, 11, 21
personal cognitive factors, **20–1**
personal observation, 4, 23
placement (social marketing), **45**, 47
planned behaviour, theory of, **15–16**
planning stage
    health promotion program, 2, **3–4**, 5
    use of theory in, 2, **3–4**, 5, **6**, 7
    see also social planning
policy change, 75
policy development, **61–74**, 75
policy influencers, 62
policy makers, 61, 62, 64
political leaders, 63

political model, **65**
political support, 6
power positions, **68**
    see also perceived power
precede/proceed model, 2
precontemplation stage (change), 17, 18
preparation stage (change), 17, 18
presuppositions, 66, 67
preventative health behaviours, 13
price (social marketing), **45**, 47
problem definition, **2–3**
problem identification, 6
problem prioritisation, 6
problem solving (community capacity), 34
problem-solving model, **65**, 66
proceed/precede model, 2
Prochaska, J.O., 16, 18
product (social marketing), 44–5, 46–7
promotion (social marketing), **45**, 47
promotion, health, xi–xii, xiii, 1, 2, **3–4**, 5, 16, 20, 22, 23, 30, **46–7**
public education campaigns, 12, 13, 23, 39, 42
public policy, xii, xiii, 7
public policy development, **61–74**, 75
public support, 6

recall, 41
receiver (communication input), **40**, 41, 47
reciprocal determinism, 20
recommendations (HIA), **72**
reinforcement, 41
relapse stage (change), 17
research, 75
    see also market research
resource mobilisation (implementation phase), **4**, 6
resources, 13, 57, 58
review (HIA), **72**
Rissel, C., 32
Rogers, Everett, 26, 27, 28, 29, 30
role models, 15, 16, 20, 23, 29, 30, 37

Rothman, J., 31, 32, 33, 36
rural communities, 28

school-based interventions, 65
scoping, **71**
screening, **70**
self-confidence, 21, 22, 23
self-efficacy, 11, 17, **21**, 23
self-initiated change, 17
settings *see* organisational
    structures
significant others, 15, 16, 41
skill acquisition, 41
smoking beliefs, 21
smoking education/cessation, 16,
    19, 20
social action, **31**, 32, 33
social capital, 36
social cognitive theory, xi, xiii, 4,
    5, **19–22**, 30
social costs, 45
social environment, 25, 62, 63, 64
social influences, 14–15, 20, 23
social marketing, xi, xiii, **42–7**
social marketing cycle, **44**
social norms, 4, 6, 16, 20, 42
social planning, **31**, 32
social pressures, 15
social structures, 25
social support, xii, 18
social variables, 40
socioeconomic values, 29
solution planning, 6
source (communication input),
    39–40, 41, 47

sponsorship, 45, 46
stimulus control, 18
subjective norms, 14, 15, 22, 23
susceptibility, 10, 11, 12
sustainability, 34, 35

tactical model, **65**
target audience, 40, 41
target market, 42, 43, 47
target variables, 4
termination stage (change), 17
theory
    definition of, **1–2**
    single or multiple, **6–8**
    use of, **2–8**
theory in practice, **75–6**
theory of planned behaviour,
    15–16
theory of reasoned action, xi, xiii,
    2, **14–16**
threat, perceived, 11
'traditional' communities, 28
transtheoretical (stages of change)
    model, xi, xiii, **16–19**
trust, 33, 36, **54**, 55, 57

understanding, 41
unemployment, 67

values, 2, 22, 29, 52
    see also beliefs

weight control, **18**, 19
Weiss, Carol, 64–5, 66, 68
workforce skills, 57